Personalised cancer medicine

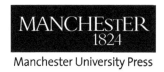

MANCHESTER
1824

Manchester University Press

INSCRIPTIONS

Series editors
Des Fitzgerald and Amy Hinterberger

Editorial advisory board
Vivette García Deister, National Autonomous University of Mexico
John Gardner, Monash University, Australia
Maja Horst, Technical University of Denmark
Robert Kirk, Manchester, UK
Stéphanie Loyd, Laval University, Canada
Alice Mah, Warwick University, UK
Deboleena Roy, Emory University, USA
Hallam Stevens, Nanyang Technological University, Singapore
Niki Vermeulen, Edinburgh, UK
Megan Warin, Adelaide University, Australia
Malte Ziewitz, Cornell University, USA

Since the very earliest studies of scientific communities, we have known that texts and worlds are bound together. One of the most important ways to stabilise, organise and grow a laboratory, a group of scholars, even an entire intellectual community, is to write things down. As for science, so for the social studies of science: Inscriptions is a space for writing, recording and inscribing the most exciting current work in sociological and anthropological – and any related – studies of science.

The series foregrounds theoretically innovative and empirically rich interdisciplinary work that is emerging in the UK and internationally. It is self-consciously hospitable in terms of its approach to discipline (all areas of social sciences are considered), topic (we are interested in all scientific objects, including biomedical objects) and scale (books will include both fine-grained case studies and broad accounts of scientific cultures).

For readers, the series signals a new generation of scholarship captured in monograph form – tracking and analysing how science moves through our societies, cultures and lives. Employing innovative methodologies for investigating changing worlds, Inscriptions is home to compelling new accounts of how science, technology, biomedicine and the environment translate and transform our social lives.

Previously published titles
Trust in the system: Research Ethics Committees and the regulation of biomedical research Adam Hedgecoe

Personalised cancer medicine

Future crafting in the genomic era

Anne Kerr, Choon Key Chekar, Emily Ross,
Julia Swallow and Sarah Cunningham-Burley

MANCHESTER UNIVERSITY PRESS

Published by Manchester University Press
Altrincham Street, Manchester M1 7JA

www.manchesteruniversitypress.co.uk

British Library Cataloguing-in-Publication Data
A catalogue record for this book is available from the British Library

ISBN   978 1 5261 4102 6   hardback

First published 2021

Typeset
by New Best-set Typesetters Ltd

Contents

Acknowledgements   vi

Introduction: Exploring personalised cancer medicine   1

1 Personalising cancer treatment and diagnosis through
   genomic medicine   22
2 Genomic techniques in standard care: gene-expression
   profiling in early-stage breast cancer   58
3 Molecular profiling for advanced gynaecological
   cancer: prolonging foreshortened futures   88
4 Optimising personalisation: adaptive trials for
   intractable cancers   118
5 Genomics at scale: participation to build the
   bioeconomy   152
6 Going private: digital culture and personalised
   medicine   183
7 At the limits of participation   211

Conclusion: Future-crafting   241

Bibliography   256
Index   271

Acknowledgements

We owe numerous debts of gratitude to colleagues, participants, advisors, friends and family who have helped us throughout our project and authorship of this book. The Wellcome Trust has generously supported our work, giving us the freedom to pursue our research ideas and involved us in a vibrant and inspiring community of academics and scholars from across the humanities and social sciences. We are particularly grateful to Dan O'Connor and Paul Woodgate for their support. Sarah would also like to thank the Rockefeller Foundation and its Bellagio Center Residency Programme which generously supported her Academic Writing Residency in the autumn of 2018. We would also like to thank colleagues and reviewers at Manchester University Press for supporting this book, particularly our commissioning editor Tom Dark.

A large project like this involves numerous colleagues who have been part of the team, including supporting it 'behind the scenes', and we want to pay tribute to their contribution here: thank you to Kay Lindsay, Gwen Jacques, Emma Doyle, Tineke Broer, Sue Chowdhry, Vivien Smith, Seiyan Yang, Mayowa Irelewuyi, Thomas Kerboul and Steph Sinclair.

Many colleagues at the universities of Leeds and Edinburgh have supported our work from its inception – thank you. Particular appreciation is due to those who provided much-welcomed advice and support throughout the project as part our Advisory Board – Debbie Beirne, David Cameron, Harry Campbell, Charlie Gourley, Graeme Laurie, Maggie Knowles, Derek Stewart, Steve Sturdy and Christopher Twelves. We are also incredibly grateful for the support of colleagues from other institutions and organisations who joined our Advisory Board – Pascale Bourret, Mary Boulton, Alberto Cambrosio and Kathryn Scott.

We have also been encouraged and supported by other 'friends to the project' who have guided our work, notably Tim Aitman, Julie Atkey, Karen Bell, Malcolm Dunlop, Tim Bishop, Sarah Chan, Sonja Erikainen, Margaret Frame, Gill Haddow, Geoff Hall, Peter Hall, Nina Hallowell, Denise Hancock, Ruth Holliday, Greg Hollin, Andrew Jack, Iain Macpherson, Julia Newton-Bishop, Martyn Pickersgill, Evi Theodoratou, Karen Throsby, Nick West, Andy Wilson, Gill Wilson, Allison Worth and Frances Yuille. We also thank our colleagues at the Cancer Research UK Edinburgh Centre and the Centre for Biomedicine, Self and Society, both at the University of Edinburgh, the Yorkshire Cancer Research, Leeds Cancer Centre and the School of Sociology and Social Policy at the University of Leeds for their intellectual and practical support.

We have benefited from warm and insightful support from our two Patient and Public Involvement panels, who have journeyed with us over the past few years, providing encouragement and very sound advice on many aspects of our research. We can't thank you enough for this.

There is a large and, at times, quite intimidating community of scholars working on cancer patienthood, and this world does not always intersect with the fields of science and technology studies and medical sociology where we ourselves are most at ease. However, we have been grateful to colleagues who have involved us in their networks, events and projects. Particular thanks are due to Alberto and Pascale, Ignacia Arteaga, Rikke Sand Andersen, Kirstin Bell, Patrick Castel, Sophie Day, Bobbie Farsides, Cinzia Greco, Henry Llewellyn, Joanna Latimer, Anneke Lucassen, Mary McBride, Mike Parker, Jeannie Shoveller, Carsten Timmermann and William Viney. Likewise, we have had the privilege of engaging with a range of clinical and scientific networks and would like to acknowledge sincerely their receptiveness to social science and to our research.

Profound and sincere thanks are also due to all of the participants in our research. Although we cannot name anyone we owe a particular debt of gratitude to a number of patients, nurses and doctors who have not only been incredibly knowledgeable and helpful participants in their own right but have also shepherded our research work so that we worked sensitively and appropriately with other staff, patients and family members. We have been humbled by the willingness of people to give time to our study, even in the most difficult of circumstances, and inspired and moved by their insightful and reflective accounts of their experiences and perspectives. At times our observations and interviews were uncomfortable and challenging, but we were continually struck by how caring participants were about these encounters and about the staff, family members and fellow patients who were part of their stories. Many patients and family members were keen to speak to us because of a sense of gratitude and reciprocity, a desire to give something back to the NHS that had cared for them, or their relatives, through their cancer. This sometimes made us worry that we had been mistaken for nurses or practitioners who deliver care or could directly influence what happens in the NHS. But through a process of dialogue and reflection in the team and with our advisors we came to appreciate these research encounters as an opportunity for dignity and self-worth for patients and family members and we accept their gift of participation with gratitude.

We write at a time of immense sadness and consternation as the world experiences a pandemic on a scale none of us could have imagined as we conducted the research reported in this book. We find it hard to know what kinds of personal or collective futures will emerge from these most difficult of circumstances, and what kind of health service and support will be available to cancer patients, given the impact of Covid-19. This pandemic brings added challenges for those with cancer, disrupting diagnosis and treatment and multiplying anxieties about the future. This is a major concern for practitioners too. We don't know what our readers will have gone through to get to this point of opening a book about personalised cancer medicine and what feelings this will generate about the topics of health and futures we discuss herein. Our best wishes and final thanks are therefore offered to you, our future readers, for taking the time to engage with our work, despite all that will have passed in the months between writing these words and the publication of our book.

Anne Kerr et al.
April 2020

Introduction
Exploring personalised cancer medicine

Personalised medicine for cancer is at the forefront of the new bioeconomy and visions for the future of healthcare. It promises treatments tailored to individuals' genomes and those of their cancers, as well as more precise diagnosis, prognosis and prevention. Widely celebrated as revolutionary and transformational, the risks and ethical conundrums of personalised medicine are confronted every day by patients, clinicians and researchers, but are consistently underplayed in the mainstream media (Marcon et al. 2018). Cancer research has a long history of optimism: the hope of living well with and beyond cancer permeates much of contemporary life. But not everyone is set to benefit from these advances in cancer medicine, and concerns about hype and over-optimism can be found across practitioner, academic and patient communities. Cancer patients, their families, policymakers, practitioners and researchers are entwined in novel practices as they navigate the promises and pitfalls of personalised medicine. In this book we investigate these practices, focusing on what is involved in promoting, receiving and delivering personalised molecular predictions, diagnoses and treatments for cancer. How is the work of crafting the optimistic or more modest and contested futures of personalised cancer medicine distributed and to what end? What kinds of value – personal, social as well as economic – are created through these practices, and for whom (Dussauge et al. 2015; Birch 2017)? How might things be organised differently to produce different kinds of values and futures for cancer patients, healthcare providers and society more generally?

Our book is based on a five-year UK-based multi-sited qualitative study of a diversity of patient, carer, practitioner, researcher, manager and policymaker experiences and accounts of genomic medicine in cancer, funded by a joint Senior Investigator Award in Society and Ethics from the Wellcome Trust.[1] We draw on a rich diversity of interviews, observations in clinics, laboratories and public events as well as textual analysis of public, policy and professional literatures and media discourses.[2] The focus of our study has been on genomics, the branch of molecular medicine concerned with mapping genomic profiles, and how this is reshaping cancer medicine and the experience of cancer. This has included diagnostic and predictive tests for cancer based on molecular profiling (shifting from single genes to panels of genes to whole genome and next generation sequencing); treatments targeted at cancers with particular molecular signatures (sometimes called tailored treatments or precision oncology); clinical trials of these new diagnostics and treatments, including new kinds of trials which offer combinations of treatments and/or adapt treatments over the course of the trial; and other research studies which gather molecular information about patients and their cancers to try to identify subtypes of cancer that are more responsive to particular treatments. We have also explored patient and public involvement in personalised cancer medicine, not just as service users or research participants, but as representatives on patient panels and other forms of involvement and engagement. Together, these activities and agendas are key parts of so-called P4 medicine, characterised as predictive, personalised, preventive and participatory (Hood and Friend 2011).

In a culture marked by enormous anticipation that biomedical innovations such as genomics may cure feared diseases such as cancer, it is hard to sound a note of caution without appearing to dash those very hopes. Maybe this can come across as a lack of compassion or even a disregard for those experiencing the disease and for those involved in their care. Our intentions could not be further from this – we want to put such experiences at the centre of our analysis because they are at the centre of personalised medicine. Yet we also want to address some of the wider, more distant processes of biomedical innovation, their drivers and their consequences. This involves unpicking how the cultural imperative to be hopeful and positive about the potential to overcome cancer, an imperative amplified by the promises offered by powerful molecular technologies, is enacted and experienced by people affected by cancer. Patients and their supporters frequently voice these hopes and obligations not only for their own, but for other patients' futures, invoking the need to extend these hopes to others. As one patient in our study commented: 'I think it's hugely exciting and I don't know if the message has entirely got across to the public out there but it's just so exciting.' Together with their clinicians, patients try out new diagnostics and drugs, take part in research, trials, fundraising and campaigns to bring this future into being. These hopes peppered our encounters with practitioners too – in the words of one oncologist: 'My hope is that by continuing to dissect the genomics [of cancer] we will come up with better treatments for specific subgroups of cancers which are genomically driven.' Being hopeful is not just an activity for the cancer clinic or clinical trial, it is part of everyday life too, marking encounters with friends and family, charitable fundraising and popular culture, where stories of the triumphs and losses of cancer are ever present. Governments, institutions, organisations and companies together with scientists, healthcare practitioners, politicians, business people and regulators also actively anticipate future benefits, including service improvements and cures as they seek to encourage participation and raise support and investment for genomic research, healthcare and bioscience infrastructure, including new molecular diagnostics and therapies for cancer. Policy discourses are replete with the language of hope and anticipation, asking us to 'welcome the genomic era and deliver the genomic dream!' (Davies 2017: 1).

These kinds of promissory discourses can be problematic for patients and professionals alike. Concerns have been raised about over-inflated expectations and harsh disappointments when test results are poor, or treatment options diminish, including when experimental and cutting-edge drugs cannot be accessed. One of the clinicians in our study clearly articulated this caution when noting, for all of the anticipation about exceptional responses, in the trial in which they are involved: 'I think that's fair to say, I mean I don't think any of the patients I've seen has had a dramatic response to date.' Frustrations with the sense of obligation always to be positive are also well documented, exemplified in feminist challenges to the 'good patient' and 'pink washed' cultures of breast cancer in particular (Ehrenreich 2001; Jain 2013; Steinberg 2015). As one patient in our study, reflecting on her experiences of being positive for family and friends fundraising on her behalf, said: 'I'm a very strong person ... but it did get to the point where I just felt like I cannot cope with this' (Stacey, see Chapter 6). Living in a culture of hope takes work and involves an emotional toll, no matter your orientation towards the promises of personalised, genomic medicine for cancer.

Traversing people's experiences and personal accounts of living with the risks and realities of cancer developing, mutating, resisting, progressing and returning and the professional work to identify, prevent and mitigate the effects of cancer in busy laboratories and clinics, we look at the kinds of futures being crafted by the actors involved, and how they interact, inflect and at other times coexist in parallel planes as genomic medicine unfolds. Our key focus is on how cancer patienthood is developing in the genomic era, including how patient identities and collectives are evolving in the context of molecular information and interventions (Clark et al. 2003; Landzelius 2006; Sulik 2009). Our exploration of performing and living 'patienthood' brings such experience into dialogue with the wider drivers of personalised medicine. This covers questions of what counts as being a 'good' or 'deserving' patient living with cancer, its risks, mutations and remissions, and how patients construct hopeful futures of cure and prevention for themselves and others, as well as the more contingent futures where foreshortened lives with cancer can be made liveable. We also explore how crafting these futures takes time, resources and care from affected individuals, families and practitioners, teasing out the strategies of maintenance, the silences, engagements and even the avoidance that this involves. This work is, at times, intense and difficult; we consider how it takes place in the context of personhood more broadly, including other kinds of life strategies, working practices and political agendas which co-produce as well sometimes overshadow or interfere with crafting personal and collective futures. The futures of patient collectives (including families and former patients), institutions and workplaces also have to be hewn alongside the work of cancer management and control, including mutations in cancer patienthood as the types and risks of cancer are stratified along molecular lines. We consider how the accounts and practices we uncover trouble narrow understandings of individual responsibility and biomedical innovation as the engine of prosperity, linking this to wider struggles around futures, democracy and value in late capitalist societies.

Future-crafting: great expectations and questions of value

More than a decade after the financial crisis, the slow growth of damaged economies and the politics of austerity in countries such as the UK have widened health inequalities and hollowed out public services. Cancer can be seen as a bellwether for late capitalist societies. Although survival rates for some cancers have improved in recent years (Arnold et al. 2019; Harrison et al. 2019), people's chances of surviving cancer vary not only according to which cancer they have but also their socio-economic circumstances. In the UK, stubborn inequalities persist and improvements in outcomes are not evenly experienced. Cancer remains a major cause of death, while estimates suggest that in the UK, 38 per cent of cancers are preventable and almost half of cancer patients are diagnosed at a late stage.[3] Incidence is on the increase, nationally and globally, due to ageing populations, with the most common cancers worldwide being lung, female breast, bowel and prostate cancer. Cancers with poor outcomes (e.g. liver, stomach) are more common in richer countries, but researchers have found that people living in poorer countries are experiencing increasing rates of cancer (Merletti et al. 2011), and there are significant differences in survival (although not incidence) depending on race and ethnicity (Ward et al. 2004). With the exception of breast cancer and melanoma, cancer is more common among deprived groups in countries such as the UK. Research in England has found that people from the most deprived areas have the highest rates of lung and cervical cancer, whereas people from more affluent areas have higher rates of breast and skin cancer (Shack et al. 2008).[4] Despite success stories due to improved treatments and prevention programmes, some cancers remain stubbornly incurable and some are less visible in research, fundraising and the media. Fear of cancer and of a lack of timely intervention are compounded by problems with health service provision, including in publicly funded systems such as the National Health Service (NHS) across the UK, which is currently experiencing severe staffing problems.[5] Improved screening and prevention programmes, earlier diagnosis, and better, more effective treatments have improved cancer mortality rates for some cancers, but services are stretched, patient experiences are diverse, and access to expensive treatments including some chemotherapy may not be available to all. Charitable fundraising for individual treatments, living costs and hospice treatment is on the increase, with patients and their families turning their leisure time and private lives over to public displays of worthiness in an effort to raise resources for targeted treatments not currently provided by the state.

The hope of personalised treatments for this most feared disease has long been part of a wider set of expectations and investments in scientific capacity and biomedical expertise in nations that have nurtured world-leading universities and hospitals as part of their global economic positioning. As countries such as the UK struggle to carve out a new economy in the face of nationalism, predatory capital and political upheaval, the bioeconomy has grown in importance. Harnessing the scientific and biomedical expertise and infrastructures of the country, particularly in the golden triangle of the south-east of England, together with the data and biological assets of the NHS, the UK has invested heavily in the genomic life sciences, with cancer a key site of collection, analysis and intervention. Working in close alliance with private capital, through a range of spin-out companies and multinationals, the UK national and devolved governments, together with major charitable funders and the expertise of the university sector, have developed an ambitious set of projects, trials, studies and initiatives to expand the new economy of personalised medicine. Patient data, tissue and other kinds of engagement and participation (for example, to improve genomic literacy), and involvement in research and uptake of services are key to the success of this new economy.

A new social contract with cancer patients is therefore emerging where their participation in research is becoming routinised as part of a drive to develop biomedical research and innovation and to improve health systems, services and patient outcomes. The vision is that patients' participation will grow the economy and secure the longer-term future of the NHS, including via special licensing and profit-sharing agreements with industry. As a result, services will become more agile and efficient, avoiding unnecessary and ineffective treatments through a more personalised approach. A focus on preventing disease rather than having to spend money on treatment will generate further savings, with the rest of the profit realised by industry contributing to national economic growth more generally. Meanwhile, individual patients are supported in their quest for tailored therapies and diagnosis through a range of experimental and cutting-edge treatments and trials. The industry, charities, advocates and carers encourage and enable patients to source new treatments, find new trials and even challenge bureaucratic decisions to extend their compromised futures. But not all patients or professionals are convinced of the logic of these investments or promised benefits, especially those who are too ill or those for whom new therapies remain beyond the horizon, only accessible for future patients, not patients in the here and now. As one patient advocate, Toni, commented about precision medicine: 'It's got everything going for it in terms of making the gap even greater between the richer and the poorer countries because these drugs, by definition, are much more expensive but they have a huge difference in their ... potential impact.' Yet opportunities and capacities to voice this kind of concern or critique are constrained by the dual promise of innovation and hope that surrounds personalised cancer medicine.

How, then, can we understand and, more importantly, intervene in these possibilities, inequalities and silences around personalised cancer medicine to craft better futures for patients, healthcare workers, services and economies? To answer this question, we need to begin with what people are currently doing – to make personalised cancer medicine work in practice – to explore what future-crafting involves and what kinds of futures are being anticipated and pursued. We need to consider how futures overlap and impinge upon each other and widen our focus from the normative vision of these biomedical developments to consider what kinds of alternative futures people carve out through their encounters with personalised cancer medicine. And we need to attend to how value circulates through these approaches and agendas – what kinds of value are being sought or achieved, and how might this be otherwise?

There are many rich and varied traditions of social scientific and philosophical literatures on which we have drawn to guide our inquiry, detailed throughout the chapters that follow. We can, however, summarise some of our key influences here, by way of introduction.

First, we are influenced by feminist and science and technology studies (STS) scholarship which seeks to change, as well as describe, the social world. This means that we aim to build on the rich description of what we have encountered in the course of our work, drawing from our findings to imagine different futures and future-crafting activities that might be cultivated as a response to our inquiry. This is not only a matter of 'putting ourselves in our story' as a reflexive ethnographic project, but of actively grappling with our own version of future-crafting. We do not do this, first and foremost, as cancer patients, or relatives of current cancer patients, but as engaged scholars with a stake in our collective futures whatever role cancer might play. As part of this engaged scholarship we have also tried to remain sensitive to the gaps, silences and omissions in our research (Haraway 1988; Puig de la Bellacasa 2011; Murphy 2012; Jain 2013), particularly the limitations in the range of voices and experiences that we have been able to document here, something we discuss further in Chapter 7. We also endeavour to reflect on our own practices of narrative as a craft – cutting, sewing, sticking, fitting, tinkering, patching data and analysis. In so doing we try to be mindful of the contingencies and relationalities, the messiness and stop–start nature of storytelling as future-crafting. This allows for the possibility of it being, at times, a relatively solitary individual practice and, at other times, a collective practice, enacted with others in one place, or across different localities and timescapes.

Second, and relatedly, we are putting patient and practitioner experiences of genomic medicine centre-stage, trying to pull together an analysis from a wide array of accounts and observations of how patients think and feel about their cancer and its treatment in the genomic era, and how practitioners keep patients in mind as they try to develop research and provide a service. We combine an interest in professional accounts and practices as well as policy approaches and agendas in an effort to understand how professional jurisdictions, epistemologies and organisations are changing in relation to personalised medicine (much of which is discussed in Chapter 1), with an interest in the complexities, tensions and contradictions of the lived experiences of patients. We are influenced by scholarship which prioritises attention to articulation work, care and emotional labour (Star 1985; James 1992; Twigg et al. 2011; Murphy 2015), work that is traditionally associated with women's devalued contribution but that is also a key part of being a patient, a provider of healthcare and a worker in the service sector. This draws our attention to the routine, mundane, everyday work of genomic medicine for cancer as a form of craft, including the intricate and skilful work of patients or practitioners that may be invisible and undervalued but is crucial to the test, treatment or research being conducted, and thereby closely linked to the work of crafting a future for ourselves and others. It also invites us to think critically about how care and other kinds of work can be experienced as neglect or inattention by others (Murphy 2015). We attend to how patient and carer identities and relationships are changing as they do some of the work of cancer research and treatment, not just as providers of data or care but as champions of new kinds of services and research, whether as representatives, campaigners or supporters of fellow patients, engaging in new kinds of 'evidence-based activism' (Rabeharisoa et al. 2014) and biosociality which forms a crucial part of the landscape of contemporary biomedicine (Rose 2001).

Third, and finally, we are focusing on futures, both imagined and made, as crafting projects rooted in practice (Adam and Groves 2007). There is a long and fascinating tradition of scholarship which investigates imaginaries and expectations as meta-discourses that perform the sociotechnical economy, establishing new markets and innovation (Hedgecoe and Martin 2003; Selin 2008; Tutton 2012; Jasanoff 2015; Brown and Rappert 2017). Medical humanities and the sociology of health and illness both have a rich seam of research on survivorship and identity-work where crafting 'culturally plausible narratives' (Frank 2003) involves embodied work in the lives of cancer survivors and the communities they come to feel responsibilities towards (see also Kaiser 2008; Kerr et al. 2019). But we know less about how contemporary cancer patients or prospective cancer patients engage with, take up or repudiate dominant expectations of prediction, personalisation, prevention and participation in this genomics era. As Michael (2017a) argues in his analysis of the enactment of 'big' and 'little' technoscience futures in which we are embroiled, there is a need to attend to how lived experiences and larger cultural and economic narratives interact. For us, these engagements, or indeed disengagements, need to be properly understood if we are really to appreciate how innovation works in practice and how it can be improved or repurposed for social good. Questions of value (Dussauge et al. 2015) are key, and here we draw on the area of valuation studies which has focused attention on the kinds of value and processes of making value that characterise all facets of contemporary working and intimate lives. In addition to understanding how economic value is produced, we want to know what other kinds of value are being made and come to light when we attend to the lived experience of innovations in the making, for recipients and subjects of research as well as professionals. This includes the value of being together with others, of feeling cared for and of worth, the value of an imagined community of other and future patients and of individual and collective meanings.

Our approach

We have tried to follow through on our commitment to lived experience, imagining other ways of generating and sharing value and attending to the craft work of future making through our own scholarship and ways of working. As a large team of researchers, we have taken on different roles and relationships to the project, the field and the writing of this book. We have also worked with others not represented as authors in this work, but whose contributions we have nevertheless sought to recognise as we write. It has been particularly important to us to write as a collective and to recognise the work of researchers who have done the bulk of data generation in the attribution of authorship for this work. At the same time, we note that we have not chosen to produce an edited collection or to attribute authorship of particular chapters as a way of delineating our contributions. Instead, we recognise that some of our team have had more of an input to specific chapters, and we have worked collectively to review and refine the analysis and writing as part of our wider collaborative efforts.

We conducted around 250 interviews with clinical and laboratory staff, patient advocates, people affected by cancer and some family members across a few UK cities between 2016 and 2019. The bulk of this fieldwork was performed by the researchers on the project (Tineke Broer, Choon Key Chekar, Sue Chowdhry, Emily Ross and Julia Swallow). This included interviews with patients and family members across five main case studies of genomic tests, studies, trials and treatments in NHS settings and private healthcare. We also carried out over sixty observations in clinics, laboratories and at public events, and a further set of digital observations across online platforms including cancer charity forums, Twitter, blogs and Facebook pages. Working with these groups and in these settings has been difficult and complex, not least because patients are often very unwell. Many of the patients we interviewed as part of our work have died, sometimes shortly after the observations or interviews took place. This brings with it a strong obligation to respectfully analyse their accounts, in all of their complexity. Cancer experiences are highly personal and emotional, and capturing the details of these experiences without intruding or causing distress is a finely balanced undertaking. Not only does it involve empathising, sensing feelings and capacities to contribute, especially knowing when to stop interactions, but it encompasses navigation of the complex institutional arrangements and representatives involved in cancer research and care. This spans the formal structures of ethical review and risk management as well as the organisational and logistical aspects of research studies, laboratories, clinics and patient pathways. It also involves working beyond physical institutions across virtual networks, to find people to engage with as part of the research, secure agreement for observations and analysis and ensure that patients and interested publics are able to shape our research agendas rather than simply act as research subjects or audiences. We had to work closely with, indeed rely upon, staff and patient advocates who acted as key gatekeepers for our study, and in so doing navigate the burdens we placed on their own time and resources, which were often stretched or in demand from numerous quarters. This included working with two Patient and Public Involvement groups we set up at the start of our research, who guided us throughout on the appropriate ways of involving and approaching patients regarding participation and in relation to the dissemination of our findings.

Our research took place at a time of crisis and worry about the future of the National Health Service after a prolonged period of low investment following the financial crisis of 2008 and an ongoing process of marketisation. It was also shaped by the cultural politics of Brexit in the UK and a growing discomfort about the politics and identities surrounding immigration, inequality and nationhood. Although this makes it a somewhat British story, it is also international in its implications and scope. We can trace the ways in which patient communities, promissory rhetoric, drugs, tissue, novel medicines and diagnostics traverse nations through our own case studies. Yet we also see many of the stories of genomics and data as national resources, and access to tests and treatments as patients' rights and responsibilities, in other national agendas and stories from patients in other countries. The complex and, at times, troubled context of the NHS clinics and laboratories made us particularly attentive to the activities and dedication of clinical and laboratory staff involved in making genomic medicine work for patients in the present and for the future.

We also became acutely aware of the gaps or absences in our inquiry as we made our way through the episodic encounters in the hospital or the community. We carried with us a strong sense of the more marginalised patients and social groups who we did not manage to speak with and include in our work, and the ever present danger that we would slip into the amplification of more articulate and insistent repertoires or 'culturally plausible narratives' (Frank 2003) as we conducted our research, as well as the difficulties of not sufficiently attending to or not being able to attend to silences, rejection and non-participation. We reflect more fully on this across each chapter and in particular in Chapter 7.

Below we detail the case studies and primary focus of each chapter, drawing out the main themes of our analysis, which we reflect upon in the concluding chapter. We briefly consider these recurrent themes here to provide a scaffold for the detailed analyses that follow and to highlight some of the implications of our work for scholarship about personalised medicine and other innovative health technologies.

First, understanding how hope operates involves grounding STS and other sociological analyses of promissory tropes in the everyday, tangled practices of personalised cancer medicine. A critical appreciation of the technoscientific promise of personalisation and attention to failures and disappointments in practice is vital, but we must also acknowledge the limits of critique, given the ways in which hopefulness around personalisation is a resource which can be taken up and reworked by embodied beings to craft liveable presents and futures. The value of critical engagement with tropes, discourses, templates and rhetoric is blunted and complicated by the messy realities of living with cancer or trying to care for those it affects. Attending to caring practices (including their limits), work, and the measurable and more diffuse kinds of care this generates has helped us to reorient our critical impulse to an appreciation of expectations as contingent, contradictory and in the making. We ask our readers and other researchers to take this complexity to the heart of their engagements with the cancer encounters we capture here and to their scholarly inquiries with patients and practitioners more generally.

Second, our research has heightened our sense of discomfort with the experiential, identity-focused work of the sociology of health and illness where documenting individual narratives and lived experience takes precedence over engagement with the institutional, political or economic processes through which experiences are lived out. Working across our case studies has made us acutely aware of the institutional structures that determine who can access or remain on these novel treatments and tests, taking us well beyond questions of survivorship as identity-work to survivorship as part of a wider political economy of material and financial resources. Medical sociological approaches to cancer crafting that are primarily concerned with identities and experiences, focusing on studies of particular types of cancer patient or community, can all too easily miss this wider terrain of patient, practitioner, carer and post- or even pre-cancer patienthood across which initiatives such as personalised medicine operate. Writing this back into their stories is a laborious and difficult process, but it is key to understanding how these technologies make their way through the world to impact patients and their carers.

Third, although we draw huge inspiration from theories and ideas of biosociality and citizenship where structures of feeling, responsibility and identity are interwoven with politics and economics, we find ourselves concerned that, once again, the focus on how experiences are organised into communities with particular subtypes or conditions does not readily fit with what we have encountered across our research, which is much more fluid and multi-layered than a focus on the molecular details of diagnostics might suggest. Patients are sometimes joined in shared agendas and pursuits in relation to their particular type of cancer, but they are often working with a diversity of other patients and allies, forming networks and collectives across molecular and bodily categories as well as across other social categories, including class and gender. We need to attend to these relationalities and the possibilities they bring for new kinds of cancer politics of solidarity in the era of personalisation, just as we must remain mindful of those patients, or groups of patients, who are excluded or marginalised from these new collective and community formations.

Fourth, welding together the different layers of engagement with personalised medicine, traversing big and little futures, also involves thinking about the work of patients, carers and researchers together, crossing laboratory, corridor and clinical spaces and moving between physical and virtual worlds where patients and their allies form networks and agendas. This process of 'moving across' settings and subjects is not a research technique that is readily accommodated by disciplinary or institutional traditions, especially ethical review or risk management, but it is vital to gathering a nuanced understanding of how personalised medicine operates at a range of levels, and, crucially, changes over time for individuals and collectives. We hope to have captured this despite the limitations of our work, and to advocate for a bolder form of interdisciplinary, ethnographic inquiry that co-researches with practitioners and patients to explore these new biomedical territories. These collaborative ways of working are vital to understanding and seeking to improve the benefits personalised medicine might bring to patients and practitioners alike.

Fifth, and finally, this study of genomics is part of a suite of social scientific and medical humanities research into innovative health technologies that have seen significant investment and interest from scientific institutions and policy actors. We have benefited from this interest and we are grateful for this support. But our study of genomics has, at times, felt like chasing a rainbow, as we switch between reading scientific and policy texts to the daily realities of the clinic, the laboratory or life with cancer. Researching with and caring for cancer patients, as well as living as best one can with cancer, certainly encompasses technological forms of personalisation and precision, but also involves navigating organisational and environmental infrastructures and barriers to care and science, work which can be relentless and at times overwhelming. We fail to capture this when we maintain a blinkered focus on the small numbers of patients – the unicorns, as one of the clinical trials assistants in our study described them – who benefit hugely from genomic personalisation. Even when we manage to capture the complexities of being part of genomic research or being on targeted treatment, we risk erasing the experiences of patients and practitioners for whom these new technologies are not available, are maybe largely irrelevant or are just one part of a wider picture of research and care. Researching genomics and other forms of personalised medicine needs to attend to all of these forms of non-participation to fully capture what these technologies mean for patients, practitioners and communities.

Book outline

Personalised medicine for cancer has many technologies, research initiatives and forms of care, including those in current practice, those in development and those anticipated. It has a variety of different meanings, interpretations and antecedents. In this book we will focus on a range of case studies of genomics and cancer that give insights into the main approaches and agendas in personalised medicine. Throughout these case studies we explore the different agendas, experiences and work involved in making the test, treatment or research trial/study work, and what kinds of value are derived in the process. We attend to the way responsibilities are distributed as futures are envisaged and enacted, how work is recognised and rewarded, what kinds of voices or experiences are discounted or absent from view, and how particular kinds of value are generated in the process. Here we add a further double P to our study of the P4 medicine agenda of which genomic medicine for cancer forms a part – *practices* of *promise* – alongside prediction, personalisation, prevention and participation. Throughout we highlight the constructed and contingent nature of these transformative agendas while also drawing attention to and at times querying their normative attributes.

Chapter 1 sets the scene for these case studies, drawing on STS and related literatures to trace the development of molecular understandings of cancer, tests and treatments and their place in the cancer clinic. The chapter covers the evolution of clinical trials and biobank research, including the rise of adaptive, basket and umbrella trials. We also explore the development of new molecular taxonomies of cancer and the implications of this fragmentation for research and treatment. The drive for personalisation is associated with new understandings of cancer as evolutionary and adaptive, and we explore how professionals make sense of this dynamism when developing treatment and understanding its effects, expressing both optimism and caution about their impact and potential. We consider the new technologies and infrastructures that genomic medicine in cancer involves, particularly in relation to tissue, data and eligibility, as well as new professional arrangements, including multidisciplinary team working, national and international consortia and public–private collaborations. We explore expert disputes, for example about the effectiveness and value of new genomic approaches, particularly in relation to the development of flexible or adaptive trials. Throughout we reflect on what these developments mean for making personalised cancer medicine work in practice, key themes in the chapters to follow.

The next three chapters form a set; they look across a range of tests, treatments and research agendas in personalised cancer medicine in NHS patient care at the time of our study. We explore personalised medicine as healthcare practice and as clinical research, beginning, in Chapter 2, with a test that is now part of standard care, moving on to consider another test that was being utilised in a small feasibility study in Chapter 3, and then to a much larger national trial of targeted treatments discussed in Chapter 4.

Chapter 2 explores the promise of prediction and prevention of recurrence in personalised medicine for some kinds of breast cancer through the case of a genomic technique already widely adopted within the UK NHS: gene-expression profiling. Although breast cancer has seen rapid advances in diagnosis and treatment, and is often cited as one of the highest-profile cancers supported by well-resourced research initiatives, it remains the most common cancer in the UK and represents 7 per cent of all cancer deaths.[6] We consider a genomic test, Oncotype DX, which seeks to identify among early breast cancer patients those who would or would not benefit from chemotherapy to prevent future recurrence. The aim here is to limit exposure to chemotherapy, which can be toxic and debilitating. The test was made valuable to the health service, practitioners and patients as a means of prediction and prevention, including via practitioners' and patients' contributions to processes of regulatory and clinical decision making surrounding the test. Considering how the test was envisaged as a benefit to the NHS and to patients in policy, practitioner and patient accounts of their experiences of decision making regarding chemotherapy, we explore how it fitted in with already complex cancer experiences and hopes for a cancer-free future. We look at how the narrative that the test offers reassurance and prediction came to dominate policy, but also consider situations where prediction and prevention were more contingent and provisional, particularly in the context of clinical encounters.

Chapter 3 explores another technique that offers personalised predictions of responses to treatments for cancer based on molecular profiling, this time for later stage gynaecological cancer patients seeking to prolong foreshortened futures in a non-curative context. Gynaecological cancers encompass cancer of the womb, ovaries, cervix, vagina and vulva and mainly affect post-menopausal women. Awareness of these cancers is low compared with other cancers such as breast cancer (in women); diagnosis and treatments and a range of campaigns and research agendas have been developed to address this. We consider a commercial test developed by a company for which we have adopted the pseudonym Virtue, not yet in routine use, that was embedded in a feasibility study in one hospital. We looked at how the feasibility study was part of building a network of collaborations and evidence to extend molecular tumour profiling in gynaecological and other cancers, and how expectations of precision and actionability were fashioned yet not always realised in practice; we focus in particular on the kinds of work this involved for practitioners and patients in the process.

In Chapter 4 we explore another route by which advanced cancer patients are offered the promise of tailored treatments that may prolong their lives, focusing on an adaptive multi-centre trial for lung cancer that aims to optimise treatments through a process of ongoing adaptation. Lung cancer has a lower public profile than some other cancers and it remains highly stigmatised because of its associations with smoking and higher prevalence among disadvantaged socio-economic groups. Concerted efforts are underway to enhance understanding of the disease and to develop new treatments. We show how the promise of the trial and targeted approaches offered a glimmer of hope for patients and practitioners coping with a bleak prognosis, exploring how the trial, treatments and patient and institutional futures were optimised in these very challenging circumstances (Montgomery 2017b). We look at how disappointments, failures and anxieties were navigated by patients and practitioners through containing scepticism backstage, calibrating expectations, including lowering (personal) expectations of extended futures (Gardner et al. 2015), and cultivating expectations that other patients will benefit in the future instead.

The next two chapters explore personalised medicine approaches that are more novel and to some extent remote from standard NHS care, but nevertheless rooted in the institutional, political and economic dynamics of UK healthcare. Chapter 5 looks at a research study of great importance to the national project of building the bioeconomy, where patients involved in cancer treatment are being recruited, but where results are unlikely to impact directly on their care. Chapter 6 looks beyond the NHS to people who are not able to get treatments that they want as part of standard care because of the regulatory and approvals process, and so are involved in raising funds or self-funding these treatments privately. These kinds of personalised medicine are therefore more innovative and speculative than the cases discussed in the previous three chapters, and as such they involve a range of pioneers and vanguards. Both chapters are set within the context of considerable inequalities in access to care and research and in the burden of cancer across different socio-economic groups (and indeed areas) in the UK, despite the public provision of a national health service which is free at the point of use. The ways the technologies are developing and are made available are shaped by the context of both austerity and marketisation of the NHS.

Chapter 5 is about large-scale national studies, recruiting patients with a range of cancers to collect extensive molecular information about cancer and ultimately inform routine patient care via precision medicine, focusing on Genomics England's 100,000 Genomes Project. After discussing the rise of these mass-participation initiatives and their strong national imaginaries of economic development and cutting-edge healthcare, we explore how practitioners, patients and families made sense of their participation, and how this related to their investment in particular institutions and futures. We explore the participatory logic of these initiatives, and the ways in which informed consent processes and genomic literacy agendas were developed and enacted to increase participation. We contrast efforts to improve genomic literacy and informed consent by clearly demarcating personal benefits in terms of improved care from the research dividend to the NHS with blurred boundaries in practice. Patients and family members were seeking care through participation and reworking efforts to improve their understanding to establish their worth as a patient and ensure optimal, personalised care into the future. We explore how this was managed by professionals to meet the aims of the programme despite their reservations about its value and implications.

While many cancer patients experience molecular diagnostics and targeted therapies as part of standard treatment or through clinical trials provided free-of-charge within the NHS, others turn to private providers to craft their own care pathways, utilising private health insurance, spending savings, taking out loans or raising money via crowdfunding online. In Chapter 6, we explore how practitioners, patients and their relatives seek to tailor their care and treatment pathways via these kinds of engagement with private healthcare. We examine the ambivalence about access to expensive experimental treatments as part of NHS or private care, and draw associations between optimisation, actionability and adaptability via personalised diagnosis and therapies and patient entrepreneurship and the intensified responsibilities for health and healthcare therein. Through this exploration we situate personalisation in relation to transformations in citizenship and consumption via social media platforms, and argue that this brings another layer of care, biosociality and identity work for patients and their relatives as they navigate the hopes and social obligations of personalised cancer therapies.

The final two chapters range across the material in the earlier chapters and bring in additional reflections about what is missing from the focus on personalisation, prediction and especially participation across our research, and in the wider public and personal narratives about personalised medicine we have been able to document. Chapter 7 considers non-participation and exclusions as well as reservation, consternation and rejections around genomic medicine in our research and in the public sphere more generally. We investigate the particular social and cultural contexts in which disengagement and resistance are generated. Exploring negative views and experiences or simply a lack of response to genomic medicine, we consider when these kinds of personalised medicine are 'not relevant to us' and why some people just do not have the capacity or resources to engage with them. Rejecting or refusing opportunities to engage with genomic medicine also results from the awareness of contested priorities such as health equality or preventive healthcare as well as a commitment to other forms of care. Not every patient can or wants to craft their own treatment pathway, or looks to the future with a sense of agency and control, and we reflect on what it means to opt out, be excluded or feel left behind by these kinds of research and care. We also discuss the ways in which different agencies and actors strive to tackle disengagement by reaching out to different communities to appeal to their sense of responsibility towards contributing to the prospects of better care for individuals and the community now and in the future. We argue that these practices present an important counterpoint to the dominant, inclusive vision of P4 medicine, particularly with regard to personalisation and participation.

In the Conclusion we draw together some broad conclusions from our case studies, reflecting on how future-crafting operates across the different groups, technologies, experiences, accounts and settings that we have explored and the kinds of work and value involved therein. We consider what rethinking and revaluing the kinds of work and futures we have encountered would mean for future research and practice.

Notes

1 Award number 104831/z/14/2 (2015–20). Ethics approval NHS REC 1 and 2 and AREA Ethics Committee University of Leeds and University of Edinburgh Usher Research Ethics Group.

2 We have anonymised interview and observational data, using pseudonyms where we draw extensively on quotes and fieldnotes involving participants, and general designations when we use quotes or fieldnotes illustratively (e.g. 'patient' or 'oncologist').

3 www.cancerresearchUK.org/health-professional/cancer-statistics-for-the-UK (accessed 22 October 2019).

4 In England cancers with the lowest five-year survival estimates are meso-thelioma (6.6%), pancreatic cancer (6.9%) and brain cancer (11.5%). Testicular cancer (96.8%), melonoma of skin (91.7%) and thyroid cancer (88.5%) have the highest five-year survival estimates (Nuffield Trust five-year cancer survival rates for adults in England between 2011 and 2015, followed up to 2016). Breast cancer is the most common cancer in women worldwide. Survival has improved due to advances in treatment,

better screening programmes and awareness. Five-year survival rates for breast cancer in UK have improved, reaching 85.6% in 2010–14.

5 The UK has good screening arrangements but when compared to other similarly wealthy countries (e.g. Japan, Australia) (see www.nuffieldtrust.org.UK/resource/cancer-survival-rates (accessed 2 October 2019)), Cancer Research UK estimates that more than 1 in 10 NHS diagnostic posts are unfilled and thousands more NHS staff will be needed in the future (see www.cancerresearchUK.org/get-involved/campaign-for-us/shoulder-to-shoulder#Shoulder_to_shoulder_across_the_UK (accessed 2 October 2019)).

6 www.cancerresearchUK.org/health-professional/cancer-statistics/statistics-by-cancer-type/breast-cancer#heading-Two (accessed 28 October 2019).

1

Personalising cancer treatment and diagnosis through genomic medicine

In this chapter, we explore how the promise and the work of personalised cancer medicine has evolved as genomic medicine has advanced. We trace some of the forms of value this has generated for patients and practitioners, industry and economies, and set the scene for our wider exploration of how this kind of future-crafting is reshaping the roles and responsibilities of cancer patients and practitioners. Drawing on a range of social scientific literatures and studies on genomic medicine for cancer, together with data from our own case studies, we discuss how patients and their families are enrolled in cancer-related genomic medicine, not just as end-users, but as co-producers of genomic knowledge and technologies. We consider how this, in turn, enacts personal and collective futures where cancer, if not cured, will be held at bay by molecular monitoring and tailored treatments.

Throughout we try to shine a light on how patients as service users, research participants, representatives, advocates, campaigners and supporters of fellow patients as well as their carers, families and friends enact, query and transform promissory visions and agendas for personalised, predictive and preventative cancer medicine through different kinds of participation (and non-participation). We trace how patients and their families engage with personalised genomic medicine for cancer through various kinds of clinical and other encounters and partnerships. We explore co-production and efforts to 'empower patients, researchers and providers to work together toward development of individualised care' in the words of the mission statement of the US NIH Precision Medicine initiative,[1] and trace the kinds of participation involved in 'participatory medicine' (Hood and Auffray 2013). As Prainsack (2017) notes, the emphasis is on patients driving these new agendas, inviting them to generate data *and* push the boundaries of research and care. Drawing on Adams et al.'s discussion of anticipation and futures, it appears that personalised medicine 'mobilizes everything and everyone', aiming for certainty but working in a context of the 'ever changing nature of truth' (2009: 256, 246).

One key area of consideration is patients' involvement in novel kinds of adaptive clinical trials that create moral, epistemic and commercial value through the continual negotiation of best possible futures for patients as individuals and as a collective (Montgomery 2017a; 2017b). We investigate the rise of 'experimental patients' in molecular oncology; patients who are actively involved in crafting treatment regimes together with healthcare professionals, including as research participants. We will also explore how patients, including potential and past patients, together with others affected by cancer in their families, act as advocates for personalised genomic medicine, particularly in relation to access to trials and costly experimental drugs, as part of these anticipatory regimes (Adams et al. 2009). Although regulatory and healthcare systems are adapting to accommodate these novel interventions, concerns about access as well as cost-effectiveness have kept the issue of cancer drugs firmly on political and personal agendas. What kinds of collective and individual actions does this bring for cancer patients and their families seeking access to novel therapies or diagnostics? How does this perform hope and anticipation about the future of personalised medicine? What kind of value does this produce and for whom?

One of the difficulties with reviewing the evolution of personalised genomic medicine for cancer is knowing where to start. Rooting the 'origin' of personalised medicine in the development of targeted therapies such as Gleevec or Herceptin foregrounds one set of technologies at the expense of other kinds of research and innovation and other kinds of practices and actors involved in these processes. The risk of a potted or so-called 'Whig' history of personalised genomic medicine for cancer is that it replicates the kinds of narratives we need to examine critically. We can think of this as the 'magic bullet' discourse – where a particular drug is given pride of place as the new cure for disease and stories are written about the heroic scientists and doctors involved in its development – a common cultural trope that can be found across policy, professional and patient accounts. To avoid replicating this, we try to offer a set of reflections on interlinked social and technological developments that form part of the story of personalised genomic medicine for cancer. We have ordered this into sections and tried to give a sense of chronology for ease of reading, but we would like to stress that we have not ranked these sections by importance. We adopt the same approach for the remainder of the book which looks more closely at a series of case studies of personalised genomic medicine for cancer.

We have also tried to exercise caution around claims to novelty. Although we can see the transformative nature of current initiatives that are driving new practices, collaborations and partnerships, we must remember that personalised medicine is not entirely new. Clinical practice has always made adjustments, for example to dosages based on the individual characteristics of patients: one size has never fitted all, even with much evidence-based medicine being driven by standard protocols (Longo 2013). So we must take care to appreciate personalised medicine as a 'rhetorical entity' (Van Lente and Rip 1998), used by actors from industry, government, regulation, academia, patient advocacy and clinical practice 'to not only describe a future state but to bring it into being' (Tutton 2012: 1721). Approaching innovation as a series of incremental shifts and reassemblages of genomic and other data, together with wider agendas of personalisation and participation, we need to attend to ideas of patient centredness, shared decision making, patient involvement and empowerment (Mead and Bower 2000; Greenhalgh 2009), as well as the integration of genomic information with an increasingly wide range of clinical, social and personal information.

Targeted treatments: a start to the story of personalised genomic medicine for cancer

Cancer came to be understood as a genetic disease in the 1980s when immunochemistry researchers began to coalesce around the so-called oncogene paradigm, approaching cancer as a subcellular disease to be treated by interfering with biochemical processes within, between and on cell surfaces. Focusing on the role of somatic, as opposed to germline (inherited), genetic mutations in stimulating the excessive growth and division of cells which formed tumours, researchers identified candidate mutations and studied the expression of proteins in patients to identify subgroups of patients with these particular genetic variations. Attention turned to blocking the action of these genes through drugs – monoclonal antibodies. These act on the genetic signalling pathway to inhibit the production of specific proteins that encourage tumour growth. What was once understood as one type of cancer became subdivided into several different subtypes (Yeo and Guan 2017). Through these developments, biomarker testing and treatment became entwined in so-called 'theragnostics', shifting the process of regulatory approval to accommodate the integration of testing technologies into treatment decisions and provisions (Fujimura 1996; Morange 1997; van Helvoort 1999; Keating and Cambrosio 2011).

As efforts intensified to identify more and more mutations with potentially actionable (druggable) pathways and to test this through ever more complex clinical trials, patients' participation in research grew. Of course, there is a long track record of patients being part of experiments in cancer medicine, but we see a shift in the scale and promise of experimentation developing over this period, as many more kinds of subtypes and targeted therapies emerged to be tried in combination (DeVita and Chu 2008; Keating and Cambrosio 2011; Jain 2013). Research became almost routinised in contemporary cancer care.

The molecular turn in cancer has deep and complex roots, but there are two paradigmatic cases that are frequently invoked as part of its history: Gleevec and Herceptin. Through telling and retelling these stories, the possibilities of personalised genomic medicine for cancer are reproduced, generating support for medical research and more permissive regulation to facilitate more of these kinds of 'wins'. Patients form an important part of these accounts, collectively and individually, as we now go on to explore.

Although Herceptin is the best-known case of early targeted therapies for cancer, scientists and social scientists have argued that it is actually imatinib (Gleevec), a small molecule that interferes with molecular pathways in chronic myeloid leukemia (CML), that is closer to a paradigm case. As Keating and Cambrosio have documented in the in-depth analysis in their book *Cancer on Trial*, Gleevec, as one of the early targeted therapies granted approval, ushered in a 'new era of therapeutic agents produced using the tools of molecular biology' (2011: 303). This development was considered revolutionary: Dan Vasella, the CEO of Novartis, the manufacturers, called his co-authored book about the drug *Magic cancer bullet: how a tiny orange pill is rewriting medical history* (Vasella and Slater 2003).

Yet, as Keating and Cambrosio (2011) demonstrate, the transformative nature of Gleevec was not just a matter of molecular pathways, but of research and regulatory processes. The trial phases proceeded rapidly and involved higher numbers of patients than usual because of a demand for participation in the context of the hope of a cure. Participants on Phase 1 trials had typically failed standard therapy but were nevertheless considered healthy enough to withstand the trial. The results were described as remarkable, with the vast majority of patients who received doses greater than 300mg going into complete remission. But there was a catch: remission was linked to continued use, thereby transforming CML into a more manageable, longer-term condition.

Phase 2 trials followed from the initial success at Phase 1 and involved high numbers of participants, achieved in part through developing an international network of trial sites and the continued involvement of Novartis in trial audit and review. Patients, too, had a role in ensuring that such research took place via the involvement of patient groups and activists. Keating and Cambrosio (2011) note that a patient petition supporting the trial was launched on the internet by a Montreal CML patient, gathering 3,000 signatures within a matter of weeks. Novartis reported receiving many letters and phone calls from patients, and their relatives, seeking access to the drug.

Subsequent Gleevec trials also saw the same kind of active patienthood, including what Keating and Cambrosio call 'epistemological activism' (2011: 340). They give the example of patients with rare gastrointestinal tumours (GIST) who organised a patient group called the Life Raft Group. Because some GIST patients had been found to be responsive to Gleevec, this kind of public patienthood focused on sharing information on trials and data on side-effects and performance. As personalised genomic medicine for cancer developed, these new kinds of patient collectives gained an increasing foothold in institutional practices such as data monitoring committees, as well as co-hosting meetings of various cancer stakeholders, in what authors such as Callon and Rabeharisoa (2008) have described as hybrid research collectives.

Gleevec was approved rapidly by the US Food and Drug Administration (FDA), less than four years after the first human dose. Its success and promise caused regulatory processes to speed up to accommodate similar innovations. Alongside these novel regulatory, partnership and trial arrangements, Gleevec also introduced a new pricing structure which saw a departure from so-called blockbuster drugs to the provision of stratified, higher-priced medicines for smaller groups of patients, so-called 'niche-busters' (Keating and Cambrosio 2011: 319).

As the GIST example illustrates, the approach taken with Gleevec is also being used for other cancers with similar molecular anomalies (Rajan 2006; Madhu 2017). Keating and Cambrosio (2011) note that these processes of redefinition were achieved in part via a proliferation of trials. By 2002 Gleevec had been part of over forty trials for a range of cancers sharing common molecular abnormalities. Gleevec also spawned a range of drug innovations. Given that a small number of patients can develop resistance to the drug, and changing the dose does not always help to manage this, this required patients to switch to other therapies. This introduces a 'proliferation of targeted agents aimed at similar pathways or receptors [which] may transform the oncology drug market' (Keating and Cambrosio 2011: 327).

Gleevec is now an established part of treatment for CML and other cancers such as gastrointestinal tumours. Patients and practitioners have come to experience some of these cancers as chronic and treatable because of these molecular actors, further motivating the promissory discourses of personalisation and cure. One of our interviewees, Andrew, who had acute myeloid leukemia, described his leukemia as a group of terrorists being fought by the British Army, with Mylotarg (a targeted therapy) described as a 'sniper', able to target abnormal cells with greater precision: 'It's actually very encouraging, it's very personalised and you think, this isn't just generic, this is to give me as an individual person the best chance of survival here.' However, other patients, who have been on targeted treatments long term, were less invested in the promise of personalisation as their treatment regimes, and indeed their cancer, became unremarkable in their everyday lives. Although one person who was on Gleevec long term considered himself 'lucky to have had that type of cancer', and to be treated with targeted therapy to which he 'responded very well', he also described feeling like a 'fraud' because of the treatment's success: 'When people say, "how's your leukemia?" it's almost like I'd forgotten I'd got it.' Others with blood cancers we interviewed were more anxious around the personalisation of treatment, expressing concern about resources. For example, one of our interviewees, Bianca, had been diagnosed with AML eighteen months prior to her interview, and had been referred urgently for treatment due to the severity of her condition. She described having a 'weird' leukemia profile, showing both a 'good' and 'bad profile' in terms of her chances of staying in remission following chemotherapy. This provoked uncertainty about her treatment plan, with the eventual decision that she undergo several rounds of chemotherapy to 'get her into remission', followed by a stem cell transplant. Bianca elaborated her mixed feelings about personalised treatment:

> I suppose in a way it gives you confidence that the treatment you're getting is as personal and appropriate for you … but … it's also a little bit kind of worrying, because you think … if all kinds of leukaemia were exactly the same would … the ability to deal with leukaemia and have a good prognosis be higher if they were only, if there was only one brand of leukaemia and you could focus everything on that, then would the outcomes improve, or because all these different brands exist and you've got to spend time dealing with all these different brands, does that mean eventual outcomes are going to be lower because resources are being spread more widely?

As this excerpt demonstrates, personalised genomic medicine sparks a range of responses from patients, from positivity to anxieties about the meanings and implications of personalisation for one's own treatment, for other patients with different profiles and about access to treatment more generally. Making sense of these various options and their implications involves patients and their families in emotional labour, working with anxiety, as well as a sense of good fortune and gratitude.

Practitioners in this field also spoke of the complex negotiation of the different kinds of treatment and research opportunities that characterised their work with patients, an ongoing process of optimisation of treatment for patients as individuals and of developing yet more personalised regimens for future patients as part of a wider bioeconomy. This involved moving between different registers of anticipation and promise, as captured in the excerpt from a senior haematologist below:

> there's a drug we use here called Ibrutinib which is a so called BTK inhibitor and that blocks or counteracts the effect of a particular mutation in leukemia cells. And in some people that works brilliantly. But you can have a mutation in another gene called CARD11 which quite commonly occurs in association with it and it just doesn't work at all ... The very first precision medicine was a type of leukemia, a drug called imatinib [Gleevec], and that worked fantastically well. And when I started off everybody who acquired myeloid leukemia died within about three or four years, and now virtually nobody dies of chronic myeloid leukemia. Now imatinib cost thirty thousand a year per patient for life, and we're going from – there's twenty-five new patients in the region a year but there's now something like five hundred people on active treatment (laughs) ... And that's just for one very rare cancer ... So there's a big economic argument here for only giving these drugs to people where it will work. But obviously the pharma companies would rather it was given to everybody (laughs). So it opens up a whole lot of areas like that as well. But at the clinical level, a lot of clinicians and patients would rather not know this, they would rather have the drug and see if it works rather than have an upfront prediction.

Here we see an account of a future of tailored medicine optimised to treat only patients who will benefit sitting alongside other accounts of tensions between providers and pharma and of patients and clinicians wanting to maintain uncertainty. This preserves a sense that their chances of success are being optimised – key themes that we will explore further throughout the book. At the same time, practitioners were also concerned about the proliferation of cancer subtypes and research activity in the blood cancer area, giving them a sense that they lacked specialisation and the capacity to deliver personalisation in a complex, ever-changing field, another key tension in our research. For example, two haematology nurses we talked with noted that the vast range of conditions meant that they are learning all the time and cannot become 'too specialised' when compared with colleagues in breast cancer care. Negotiating professional status and expertise was an integral part of delivering these new opportunities and future possibilities for patients.

Patients are part of the Gleevec story as research subjects, advocates and beneficiaries, but as our own research demonstrates, their experiences of personalised treatments are more wide ranging and complex than the optimistic stories of magic bullets or even epistemological activism might suggest. We can identify similar patterns with Herceptin, arguably an even better-known exemplar of transformative personalisation, as we now go on to discuss.

Herceptin's story is a key part of the success narrative of personalised cancer medicine, eclipsing Gleevec in the public imaginary, not least because of the gender health politics surrounding breast cancer research and care (see Hedgecoe 2004; Abelson and Collins 2009; Keating and Cambrosio 2011). It was developed after scientists at the National Cancer Institute in the US found that a mutation in HER2 (Human Epidermal Growth Factor Receptor 2) could cause normal cells to grow uncontrollably and that the gene's protein was over-expressed in around 30 per cent of breast cancers. It was subsequently shown that an antibody specific to HER2 could slow the growth of breast cancer cells in the laboratory. University scientists went on to collaborate with Genetech, a company that is widely regarded as the pioneer of biotechnology, to develop a HER2-specific antibody called Trastuzumab (Herceptin). In the 1990s, trials of Herceptin, in combination with chemotherapy for patients with metastatic cancers, showed positive outcomes, increasing the median survival rate for patients on a combination of Herceptin and chemotherapy by five months as compared with patients on chemotherapy alone. It was first licensed by the FDA in 1998, for use in patients with metastatic breast cancer, and subsequently approved in the UK in 2002. Use was extended quite quickly, from a treatment for metastatic breast cancer (on its own or in combination with a specific chemotherapy, paclitaxel) to a treatment for early-stage breast cancer. Roche, which acquired a major stake in Genetech in 1990, successfully sought to extend Herceptin's licence to include early-stage breast cancers, and in 2006 the FDA licensed the drug for use with a combination of chemotherapies (doxorubicin, cyclophosphamide and paclitaxel) as an adjuvant treatment for patients with early-stage (localised) HER2 positive breast cancer after surgery. Herceptin became Roche's fifth highest-selling drug by 2002 (Hedgecoe 2004), worth £460 million, and led to a 20 per cent increase in Genetech profits. Herceptin also heralded the 'package' approach to test/treatment that persists today. Roche funded HER2 tests before the drug was approved, thus ensuring that it became embedded in oncology practice, preparing a pathway for the drug once it was approved.

As with Gleevec, patients feature in the story of Herceptin as advocates, especially as lobbyists for extending the licence of this treatment to early-stage breast cancer via a concerted media campaign. There is a strong history of advocacy among breast cancer patients, including grassroots movements such as Breast Cancer Action in San Francisco Bay in the US (Klawiter 2004) through to large-scale commercially funded breast cancer awareness campaigns (Sulik 2014). This kind of advocacy presaged a more institutionalised role for patient involvement as well as contributing to the high profiles of breast cancer and breast cancer experience that have shaped public discourse of cancer, including around survivorship, access to drugs and prevention and early detection.

Abraham (2009) highlights the alliances with patients and patient organisations that were involved in the promissory agendas around Herceptin, noting that Roche reputedly engaged public relations companies to encourage women to campaign for access to the drug, including in the NHS in the UK, in so doing constituting its own version of engaged and optimistic patienthood. A 2006 BBC report by Sanchia Berg[2] described the experience of the late Professor Lisa Jardine, professor of history, public intellectual and former chair of the Human Fertilisation and Embryology Authority, who was contacted on behalf of Roche to assist with her accessing Herceptin prior to NICE approval. Although Jardine was reportedly alarmed by this PR exercise and did not enter into an arrangement with Roche, the report noted a number of cases covered in the national media of women who had early-stage breast cancer and whose Primary Care Trust (PCT) had refused funding for Herceptin, with the emphasis on trying to 'shame' trusts into funding the treatment. Herceptin, and the associated test for HER2, was subsequently approved by NICE for early-stage breast cancer, but questions were asked about the involvement of Roche in these media cases and about the speed of the decision, which appeared to be rushed according to some commentators in the Berg report, including Dr Richard Horton, the editor of *The Lancet*.

Supportive press coverage featuring patient testimony is a feature of these campaigns for extended access. In a comparative analysis of UK and Canadian coverage of Herceptin, Abelson and Collins (2009) found that reporters presented individualistic perspectives on access to Herceptin as highly beneficial. This is echoed in a paper on the New Zealand context by Gabe et al., in which they describe coverage as being dominated by 'personal stories drawing on the news frame of "desperate, sick women in double jeopardy because of callous government/incompetent bureaucracy"' (Gabe et al. 2012: 2358, quoting MacKenzie et al. 2008: 305). As Gabe et al. (2012) note, press coverage is shaped by press releases from companies and, in the case of Herceptin, Roche used this route effectively as part of its campaign for approvals. For example, a Roche press release covering the interim results of trials of Herceptin in early-stage breast cancers, apparently timed to coincide with the American Society for Clinical Oncology meeting in June 2005, noted that 'women with early stage HER-2 positive breast cancer reduced their risk of their cancer returning by 46 percent when using the targeted therapy Herceptin' (Gabe et al. 2012: 2355, quoting Roche press release).[3] Patient narratives, while providing a window on to the experience of cancer and all its hardships, can also be deployed strategically by pharma to garner support and demand. Indeed, individual cases and stories fit well with the individualising paradigm of personalised, precision medicine, providing authenticity through personal experience and individual successes and efforts. But patient groups can become assimilated in other kinds of campaigns too. Gabe et al. discuss the example of the Breast Cancer Advocacy Association in New Zealand, which lobbied regulators and government to improve access, including supporting a 2008 court case by a group of 'Herceptin Heroes' which resulted in the regulator having to conduct further consultation to formulate policy. Through these practices the side-effects of drugs such as Herceptin, which include, among others, cardiac toxicity, are downplayed in favour of its promise of longer lives for patients.

As with Gleevec, new multinational consortia were developed to establish viable trials for the drug. HERA (HERceptin Adjuvant) was initially run by the not-for-profit Breast International Group, established in 1996 and supported by Roche. As Keating and Cambrosio (2011) discuss, this 'consortia of consortia' encompassed numerous groups, hospitals, laboratories and centres, together with a patient organization, Europa Donna, which were represented on the trial committee. The complex arrangements for data governance and trial management, designed to maintain 'scientific independence' from industry, led to tensions with Roche, and careful configuration of data monitoring committees was required to maintain their collaboration (Keating and Cambrosio 2011: 329). The 'molecular turn' challenged a trial methodology already under strain as patients and clinicians sought out novel treatments and changed assessment criteria to demonstrate therapeutic benefit. Later trials designed to assess the efficacy of Herceptin also ran into difficulty as clinicians were reluctant to assign patients to the option when Herceptin was discontinued.

It is well established that clinicians and scientists worked closely with the manufacturer of Herceptin to gain approval for the drug through research trials and other studies. Gabe et al. (2012; see also Busfield 2006; Light 2010) give an example of this kind of co-production, which features a review of Herceptin in the clinical setting by breast cancer researchers from Guy's and St Thomas's Hospital, London (Miles 2001). Although the author acknowledged support from industry, including Roche, Gabe et al. (2012) note that industry support is not mentioned in other papers, including a supportive review of recent trials, methods of HER2 testing and the combination use of Herceptin.

Patienthood in media and corporate narratives of Herceptin is framed in familiar registers of hope and despair. But as other social research demonstrates, the take-up of Herceptin, and patients' and practitioners' roles therein, was more complex and their attitudes were more ambivalent than these versions of patienthood suggest. Even though HER2 was one of only several targetable mutations where there was consensus about its predictive and prognostic value (it is now a routine test for invasive breast cancer in the UK), professionals were wary about the gap between the messy realities of treatment and patient expectations as it was introduced into practice (Tutton and Jamie 2013). Hedgecoe's (2004; 2005) detailed work on the development of pharmacogenomics in a UK breast cancer clinic in the 2000s explores these themes. Hedgecoe observed how metastatic breast cancer patients could be tested for HER2, and Herceptin was offered to HER2+ patients (provided free by Roche), but he notes that clinicians did not rush to test but sought to protect patients from information overload. In the words of one of Hedgecoe's interviewees, it is only 'At the point at which you can do something about it, then it [HER2 testing] becomes more relevant' (Hedgecoe 2005: 1204). Hedgecoe draws attention to other kinds of clinician ambivalence around HER2 testing in the UK at this time, including in comparison with practice elsewhere, notably the US, where, in 2001, the American Society of Cancer Oncology recommended that HER2 testing be available to every primary breast cancer patient. He links UK clinicians' reticence to view HER2 as 'special' to a general culture of keeping expenses down as compared to other healthcare systems. Clinicians' concerns about managing patients' expectations and dealing with disappointments (when HER2 over-expression was not detected and Herceptin was not prescribed) increased their ambivalence about the test.

Patients also experience ambivalence about this kind of testing, even now that it is well established. Although many of the social scientific and popular narratives of Herceptin have focused on the activism for access to the drug in which some patients became involved, this kind of patient activity is not all that being on or accessing Herceptin involves. A particular issue arises here regarding being a HER2+ subtype patient entitled to Herceptin. Breast cancer patients must negotiate these kinds of typologies, and the resultant stratification of treatment experience, with their friends and other people they meet, as the excerpt below from an interview with Jane, in her early fifties, who had had cancer at a relatively young age and was on maintenance medication, illustrates:

> There's sort of the public perception is … there is just breast cancer and I thought that, but there isn't, there are very different types and it can be very individual so … that's sometimes quite hard when other people ask you about it, to try to say, well, I didn't have the same thing as your mum.

'Not being the same' can introduce anxiety, doubt and concern, given that it can mean not accessing particular or familiar kinds of treatments like others. Another person with breast cancer who we interviewed, Yvette, described how she was offered surgery first, whereas her friend, another breast cancer patient with a popular blog, was receiving neoadjuvant chemotherapy before surgery (the patient pathway for cases of triple negative or HER2+ cancers or for those women with larger tumours [Derks and van de Velde 2018]). This made Yvette wonder 'why am I not getting that?'; she speculated about whether this was because her friend was receiving private healthcare, telling us that she did not understand 'how they make those decisions'.

When we delve deeper into experiences of Herceptin and HER2, we find that breast cancer patients and practitioners, like blood cancer patients and practitioners using targeted treatments such as Gleevec, have a range of experiences of personalised genomic medicine for cancer that include, but also go beyond, the roles of enthusiastic research beneficiary or advocate. Patients and practitioners are weaving genomic medicine into their encounters with other patients, relatives, tests and treatments as they navigate their future and that of others. This involves a complexity of values and work, as we go on to explore further below. Here, patienthood begins to multiply as experiences and representations proliferate and diverge, but it also converges in dominant media and corporate tropes of active, engaged and sometimes desperate patients.

Targeted therapies proliferate

The promise of a suite of targeted therapies to give patients and clinicians more options to treat cancers as they resist, mutate and evolve over time is a powerful feature of personalised cancer medicine. As a recent report from the Institute of Cancer Research on improved access to targeted therapies asserts:

> Cancer is enormously complex, and it can adapt and evolve in response to changes in its environment – including drug treatment. Only through radical innovation will we deliver the step-change improvements we need in cancer treatment, by attacking cancer in new ways that allow us to overcome or prevent drug resistance. We need to create a wider variety of targeted drugs and immunotherapies and find new treatment combinations that can block cancer's escape routes.[4]

Popular culture and everyday talk is replete with personal stories of struggles around access, scientific breakthroughs and big futures of cancer as a chronic, treatable disease. We can trace these narratives across professional, popular and policy literatures, our own observations and interviews, much of which hinge on the idea of the drug as a potent force in the ongoing battle against cancer in both the body and the body politic. In this cultural narrative the next drug is always around the corner; radical innovation becomes routine, as one lung cancer consultant explained in relation to news of a recent approval:

> And quite excitingly, just in this week … one of those drugs has just been NICE approved, … as a follow on treatment for patients who've stopped responding to the first tablet. So when you stop responding to the first tablet … instead of having to go and have chemotherapy you can go and have another tablet which … is targeted as well. So that gives you hope that you might then find a third tablet and a fourth tablet when they stop responding to that.

Many patients are already able to access tried and tested therapies such as Gleevec and Herceptin, but for other patients with different kinds of cancer, including lung cancer patients, drugs are more experimental and less readily accessible. In the UK, accessing drugs can involve making a case for exceptional or compassionate use, or joining a trial. It can also involve challenges to NHS trusts, NICE decision making and efforts to raise funds privately. For advanced or metastatic patients in particular, targeted drugs which offer extra months of life with symptoms held at bay are highly valued. However, for health systems, methodologies that determine efficacy based on a range of factors including quality of life, balancing wider public benefits through effective allocation of healthcare resources, mean that these benefits are not always sufficient to warrant approval. This has led to a series of disputes around access to tailored therapies, for example Avastin (for ovarian and colorectal cancer) and Kadcyla (for breast cancer) in the UK, with some patients turning to charitable fundraising or private funds to access these and other drugs. These campaigns can have a considerable media profile, giving a sense that these activities are both common and necessary, intensifying a media discourse of the NHS as failing to provide. This has enrolled patients in campaigning for access alongside others affected, as well as relatives and other advocates, something we discuss in Chapter 6. For example, with regard to a recent campaign for access to

Avastin by a cervical cancer patient who had been denied treatments available in England but not in Wales, ITV news quoted the patient: 'I feel very angry about it, it's so unfair – this is playing with people's lives. But I'm fighting it for others both in England and Wales, and for those who are too afraid to speak out.'[5] Patients seeking access to these kinds of treatments also have to navigate personal networks and complex healthcare provision, including sometimes predatory markets, as Keir, a campaigner for better drug access for cancer and other patients, described:

> there are certain circumstances where ... crowdfunding [is for] a medically reputable drug ... But it's horrendous that patients are being forced to take that, it's a hugely stressful undertaking for them. They're trying to do crowdfunding, they've got neighbours who are ... running charity events ... they've got to ... give a huge amount of themselves to try and thank everybody, and engage everybody to try and get enough money in the door, on top ... managing cancer treatment ... trying to do their day job, and continue to bring up their kids ... that is a real ... system failure.

Uncertainties, doubts and disappointments have also proliferated alongside these drug developments and campaigns for access. As practitioners in our research often attested, cancer is complex and ever-changing, and drugs rarely deliver the kinds of benefits seen with the paradigmatic cases of Herceptin or Gleevec, as this oncologist describes:

> No, no targeted therapy has yet made otherwise incurable metastatic cancer curable. What they have done has meant that in the same way that chemotherapy can prolong survival from six months to two or three years in breast cancer or bowel cancer, there are now diseases like melanoma and renal cancer where previously chemotherapy didn't have a role where now patients can live two, three, four, sometimes longer. But they are only seeing results akin to what we see in breast cancer with hormone therapy or with Herceptin.
>
> So ... they haven't been the, the sort of paradigm shift ... which we had hoped they would be ... fifteen years ago ... the way these drugs were sold was that they were going to take cancer and turn it into a chronic disease, like hypertension or like diabetes ... [this] a huge new era hasn't materialised. What instead we're seeing is a new generation of drugs, sometimes but not always ... less toxic than chemotherapy that, that add to the armamentarium of treatment that

we have, but haven't had that effect of, of, of meaning that people live ten, fifteen, twenty years, whereas previously they, they would only have lived a few weeks or months. They now live for many months or a few years, rather than several months or a year.

And do you think patients understand this?

I think patients' expectations of ... cancer treatments generally are ... are over-optimistic.

These concerns are echoed across professional and social scientific literatures. Social scientists such as Davis (2015) have argued that patients' overestimation of the benefits and underestimation of the toxicity of these treatments is a systemic problem rather than a feature of individual patient-clinician decisions. For Davis, permissive regulatory environments, government promotion of bioscience markets as a vehicle for economic growth and national competitiveness, and close ties and connections between industry, oncology, government and patient organisations have fuelled a culture of overtreatment, as have scientific and media reporting and medical practice intent on maintaining hope in the fight against cancer. As Davis notes, 'Publication bias, distorted scientific reporting, promotional material, and stories of "miracle" drugs percolate against a background discourse of "science at a crossroads" and "new eras"' (2015: 213).

We must nevertheless recognise that patients are not simply dupes of this promissory bioeconomy. Instead they are active participants in its articulation and contestation. Patients in our study were by no means predominantly pessimistic nor wildly optimistic but, instead, were often strategic and nuanced in their engagement with these new therapies. Even patients funding treatments privately had a careful analysis of why they were taking this approach. Phil, a patient with advanced bowel cancer who was self-funding Avastin, explained:

look, you know, I'm in a situation where I've got advanced bowel cancer ... I can afford to do it, fortunately, so I thought ... although it's expensive ... I'm going to ... give it a whirl. ... I don't want to ... die wondering whether ... it would've made a difference or not.

Others told us how they had accepted not being able to access targeted therapies. Alison, a patient advocate in her mid-sixties who had previously worked in special education, who had experienced pancreatic and breast cancer, described her philosophy thus:

> Now my brother works for [a pharmaceutical company], he used to work for them in America. He says 'we've got a new drug' but we spoke to the surgeons here, I couldn't do it because ... it hadn't been passed [by the regulator] so nobody could administer this drug, they had great success. [My brother] got all my test results, he said 'right, you have a very rare type of pancreatic cancer ... and this drug seems to be working'. So he speaks to the oncologist [who says], 'No you can't do it because it's not licenced.'
>
> So I went 'that's fine' ... things happen in life for reasons, ok ... it's part of our journey ... it wasn't for me ... It's like ... if you're buying a house or something and you miss out on it, it wasn't meant for you, don't worry or stress about it ... What's meant for you, will happen and it might be even better.

Alison told us how her family rallied around her when she experienced her first cancer. Her daughter, a veterinary nurse specialising in cancer, made time to pick her up after her appointments, while her husband sought out second opinions and support networks. Drawing on their social and cultural capital, cancer patients and their families navigate the stage and subtype of their cancer and access to treatments that might extend their future. This not only involves building from and troubling cancer identities of survivorship and developing novel campaigning tactics and alliances, but it incorporates more ordinary ways of living with uncertainty and hope. Through these kinds of activities and other reflections, patients, relatives and practitioners come to terms with the opportunities and setbacks of personalised genomic medicine for cancer, even as they might also articulate other, much more overt promissory discourses elsewhere. These themes cut across the chapters to follow and are explored in particular depth in Chapter 6.

Personalising prognosis, prediction and diagnosis

Effectively targeting treatments relies on molecular markers; together they are reconfiguring how cancers are classified (Nair et al. 2018). New molecular markers, disease categories and targeted treatment options are part of a nexus rather than a linear process of discovery and intervention. This means that prognostics, prediction and diagnosis, always rather dynamic in the context of cancer, are becoming even more so, as genomic tests and assays provide ever more data on a patient's risks, mutating tumour and responses to treatment. Diagnosis and therapy 'bleed into each other' as Bourret et al. (2011) note, transforming clinical decision making as the results of genomic testing rework established understandings and practices.

In addition to molecular subtypes of blood and breast cancers, as discussed above, there are now a range of established molecular markers of other cancers such as colon, lung cancer, ovarian and melanoma. For example, colorectal cancers can be classified according to five biomarkers including KRAS. Particular mutations can also be found in different kinds of cancers; for example, the KRAS mutation has been identified in colon and lung cancers, and the BRAF mutation has been found in colon cancer and melanoma. As treatments are increasingly guided by molecular profiling, not just the location of cancer in particular areas of the body, professionals have begun to discuss a new paradigm of diagnosis and classification based on such molecular markers, as in the excerpt below:

> It is the mutation-guided therapeutics, rather than the traditional cancer type-dependence classification, such as that based on classical anatomy and histology, that has etched a new context ... This concept has compelled a paradigm shift. Now patients with BRAF V600E mutations would be prescribed the same drug regimen irrespective of their cancer type and location, for example, acute myeloid leukemia, breast cancer, or melanoma. (Nussinov et al. 2019)

Cancer has traditionally been diagnosed histologically, through the microscope. Serum markers such as the prostate antigen test (PSA) were subsequently developed for monitoring those with or at risk of cancer. This focus on biomarkers was also brought together with advances in the understanding of oncogenes and tumour-suppressor genes and genomic technologies to develop a range of biomarker companion tests for proteins associated with specific subtypes of cancer, such as HER2. The successes of Gleevec and Herceptin were promising, but in fact the complexities of cancer are such that there is rarely only one gene of central importance in its development, and testing moved towards looking at groups or clusters of molecular biomarkers that would assist with defining and, crucially, predicting the course of the disease or the usefulness of one particular drug, not least to avoid ineffective treatment. Gene-expression profiling has developed to identify patterns within cancer tumours and this has led to the identification of subtypes based on these patterns for cancers such as leukemia and breast cancer. This has developed into a range of tests to aid treatment decision making, particularly for breast cancer, many of which are commercially available and based on proprietary algorithms. MammaPrint® (Agendia, Amsterdam) was one of the early multi-gene panel tests to be approved by the FDA in 2007 to predict breast cancer relapse. Oncotype DX® (Genomic Health, Redwood City, CA) is also used to predict the risk of recurrence of certain kinds of breast cancer in order to aid treatment decisions, as we go on to discuss in Chapter 2. Cambrosio et al. have written about how these tests were developed by scientific and commercial partners in concert with evolving regulatory arrangements, 'forming heterogeneous assemblages that seek to singularize treatments' (Cambrosio et al. 2019: 2).

Novel molecular tests are particularly interesting because they involve rearrangements of private–public relations, pathology and clinical decision making around prognosis and prediction (Kohli-Laven et al. 2011). For example, MammaPrint and Oncotype DX were developed in company laboratories to which clinicians must send samples for analysis. Results are returned in the form of reports of likelihood or risk of recurrence to form part of a broader set of results from other non-molecular tests and other information that clinicians use as part of clinical decision making. The roles of hospital-based and regional pathology services are also reconfigured through the development of oncogene sequencing, both in-house and externally, resulting in tensions and threats to professional autonomy that have to be managed. This includes pre-screening to identify low-risk cases where proprietary testing might not be cost-effective (Dabbs et al. 2018; Beaudevin et al. 2019). As Nelson et al. have argued, these genomic tests, together with the therapeutic regimes they invoke, are part of a new paradigm of 'actionability' in cancer which is transforming alongside trial arrangements, regulatory processes and healthcare, where the 'articulation of molecular hypotheses and experimental therapeutics become central to patient care' (Nelson et al. 2013: 413). They note, however, that this brings uncertainty about how to make meanings from molecular results: actionability is thus an 'experimental space' where different approaches and interpretations coexist and must be resolved in the 'knowledge architecture of clinical oncology' (Nelson et al. 2013: 413).

Within this space, clinicians and patients must also engage with molecular results about cancer as another layer of information that has to be analysed, interpreted and considered in relation to other aspects of the patient's disease, including lifestyle, emotional state and social location, and their capacity and appetite for further treatment. Making a genomic test valuable as part of their decision making includes making sense of intermediate or 'grey areas' and crafting reassurance or managing the anxieties that ensue. Patient experiences of tests using biomarkers (not genomic technologies) highlight some of the intricacies of these processes. Bell and Kazanjian's (2011) research on PSA, a molecular marker which is used to monitor the risk of prostate cancer developing, progressing or returning, shows how the responsibility to be well is managed by patients and practitioners through engagement with these results. Although its effectiveness as a screening or monitoring tool is highly contested because of questions about its predictive value (Bickers and Aukim-Hastie 2009), its continued use in some contexts can be explained by neoliberal governance whereby individuals become responsible for identifying and minimising their risk of disease (Petersen and Lupton 1997). Bell and Kazanjian (2011) show how men experiencing the test had to navigate considerable anxiety and uncertainty, together with expectations of action from family members and clinicians as part of the process of being responsible. They argue that molecular measures intensify a sense of living with cancer even when results suggest lower risks, echoing the findings of Hamilton's (1999) study of women's experiences of CA-125 biomarker monitoring for recurrent ovarian cancer, another contested measure that lacks sensitivity and specificity. Quoting from Hamilton, Bell and Kazanjian note:

> Many women begin to identify their CA125 levels of the evidence of disease status. If it is low, they feel relieved and in control … If the level is elevated from prior levels, they know the disease is back and must plan for more treatment. Unfortunately, even normal insignificant

fluctuations in CA125 levels take on enormous meaning. As a result, emotional well-being may come to depend on lower CA125 number, even if numbers remain in the normal range. Patients may find themselves on an 'emotional roller coaster' with ups and downs determined by the direction of serum blood levels. (Bell and Kazanjian 2011: 193)

In later work, Bell goes on to note that this sense of what Gillespie (2012) has called 'measured vulnerability' can be intensified by molecular biomarkers, whereas for other patients these results do provide reassurance because of 'the semiotic potency of biomarker numbers as transparent, material indices' (Bell 2013: 230) in the context of ongoing uncertainty and fear around cancer.

Results such as these nevertheless create a space for patients to negotiate the meaning of their illness and treatment arrangements with their clinicians, 'empowering patients to challenge physician decision making – especially in circumstances where physicians are seen to be overly passive or nihilistic' (Bell 2013: 139). Genomic results add a further layer of complexity to these processes, promising more precise personalisation but also requiring work to make sense of results in a responsible manner. Our analysis of personal blogs and online forums discussing Prolaris (Yan 2017), a gene-expression profiling test to support therapeutic decision making for prostate cancer by predicting a tumour's potential aggressiveness, suggests that the responsibility to be positive is powerful. Men crafted 'peace of mind' through their engagement with the test, even when the results were negative or unwelcome indicators of foreshortened futures. These positive registers of responsible patienthood were reinforced in company blogs and through virtual patient networks which together advocated for genomic testing as a means of patient support.

As molecular profiling to determine treatments matures and expands through the use of genomic technologies, many more patients with or at risk of cancer developing or returning will be drawn into this kind of work, managing uncertainty and the anxieties it can provoke, finding reassurance and making meaning out of test results with clinicians and/or other affected individuals they encounter in face-to-face and online support groups. Here they are crafting identities and futures together, seeking to realise value from tests in the process. Patients actively seeking access to tests might also be drawn into regulatory decision making, just as with targeted treatments, perhaps working with industry, charities and/or clinicians and scientists as these experimental spaces become more mainstream. This involves crafting bigger futures and engaging in valuation work for industry and government, whereas for other patients who are less engaged, active or well, future-crafting takes place on a much more local scale. We go on to explore this further in Chapters 2 and 3 where we focus on two very different tests and scales of future-crafting, work and value making for breast and gynaecological cancers.

Adaptive trials

Since the development of Herceptin and Gleevec a whole host of molecular markers and targeted therapies for cancers have emerged. Among these are therapies which target the BRAF mutation in metastatic malignant melanoma (Vemurafenib), the EGFR mutation in non-small-cell lung cancer (Erlotinib and Gefitinib) and the KRAS mutation in colorectal cancer (Cetuximab). Similar to the stories of Herceptin and Gleevec, these therapies emerged through complex trial and organisational arrangements, including the involvement of public–private partnerships, international collaboration and patient groups. Participation in trials for other targeted therapies, or combinations of therapies, has become a more common expectation for cancer patients, as has access to experimental drugs (although trials and drugs are not accessible for all patients, as this depends on their health, prior treatment, type or stage of cancer as well as genomic-based eligibility). This involves patients and their advocates in a range of activities to understand, source and secure particular treatments or combinations of treatments through being on trial, as access to personalised therapies becomes an expected part of the patient journey, reinforced by the promise of personalised cancer medicine.

Cambrosio et al. (2018) stress the importance of understanding this 'reshuffling' of the research/care distinction and new forms of 'experimental care' that have emerged in personalised cancer medicine. This draws our attention to the care enacted and received by patients while on clinical trials which are increasingly adaptive or novel in other respects (for example, umbrella and basket trials which bring patients together based on their molecular profile, not their cancer types), as well as experiments in care that take place beyond involvement in trials through a culture of 'trial and error' approach to treatments. The world of targeted treatments is one of novel combinations, unknown side-effects, tumour heterogeneity, resistance, adaption and evolution. Patients, together with family members, clinicians and scientists, are researching together as they navigate the meanings and possibilities of molecular diagnostics and therapies. This is no longer simply testing and treating accordingly in a linear fashion, but treating and profiling in iteration, adapting treatments and, increasingly with the development of so-called liquid biopsies that test circulating tumour DNA (avoiding the need for invasive biopsies), retesting as a form of theranostics. Research is also becoming embedded in care through architectures such as the SHIVA[6] trial's Molecular Tumour Boards and other larger-scale infrastructure such as cohort management systems that have remained in place after the trials have ended as a means of integrating research and care more routinely through directing patients to trials and/or novel experimental treatments as part of their care:

> The body of the patient becomes simultaneously a locus of experimenta-tion and the subject of hopefully more effective (because more precisely tailored) care. To put it in a slightly different way, experimentation on an individual patient also qualifies as a form of personalized care. (Cambrosio et al. 2018: 218)

Together, these new practices are reconfiguring patients' and profes-sional and institutional futures. Hopeful futures of remission and even cure are cultivated alongside visions of more efficient services and responsive professionals. These promissory big futures are enacted in trials and experimental treatments. But other kinds of more provisional and, at times, unwelcome futures remain in play, as the complex realities of vulnerable bodies and institutional processes emerge and impinge on these processes.

As well as being built around a multi-drug regimen, these new trial arrangements rework assessment criteria to demonstrate thera-peutic benefit. As Keating and Cambrosio (2011: 365) note, this involves new 'end-points' such as 'disease stabilization, time to progression and progression-free survival' for phase 2 and 3 trials, reworking goals for the future in the process. It is also worth noting here that although randomisation is common in other trials, this has always been controversial in cancer, and the genomic era has involved an acceleration of new trial designs which do not involve randomisation. Keating and Cambrosio (2011) note that a general feature of these kinds of trials is that they are not statistically robust, tending to involve small numbers of patients and a lack of ability to compare targeted therapies such as Herceptin with other combination therapies, thereby tending to bias findings in favour of Herceptin-based combinations. Adaptive trials are part of the experimental process, rather than a fixed methodology to be applied routinely, and the nature of supporting evidence is co-produced in a clinical context where the promise of the drug holds great sway.

The changing nature of trials and issues over access and efficacy have not only drawn more patients into experimental practices as part of their treatment, they have also sparked international debates around measures of success and clinical trial design, as well as the processes for approval based on clinical effectiveness in which trials play a crucial role. Trial design, pricing structures and measures of efficacy of tailored, precision or stratified cancer medicines are all areas of flux at the present time, generating public doubt about the promise of personalisation and its role in cancer care now and in the future. This has taken the form of controversy around the extent to which precision or personalised medicine is worthy of the celebration and expectations in popular and professional discourses about its possibilities. Borad and LoRusso list some of the problems with establishing benefit in this area as follows:

> selection bias present in single-cohort studies lacking a control arm, ascription of success to alterations being identified simply as actionable (instead of more rigorous criteria that would classify alterations as useful or not on the basis of strength as a predictive marker for therapeutic efficacy), or leading to change in therapy (irrespective of such a change producing a favorable outcome), heterogeneity of histologic tumor types, and inflation of value of broad-based NGS profiling in the setting of inclusion of patients with well characterized alterations (e.g., patients with BRAF V600E melanoma) in reported studies. (2017: 1583)

As the authors go on to discuss, the SHIVA trial mentioned above is an oft-cited example of the difficulties with researching precision medicine. The first SHIVA trial did not find any benefit in therapies allocated on the basis of genomic profiling as compared to therapies allocated using conventional clinical decision-making tools. A second SHIVA trial is, however, ongoing and, despite the problems with the first trial, SHIVA has been hailed as a success in clinical trial design because it did suggest that targeted therapy based on profiling might be a valid approach in a subgroup of patients with a particular kind of molecular alteration.[7] The lack of definitive proof of benefit from (randomised) trials has been taken by some critics as evidence that personalised or precision medicine is over-hyped. One haematologist, Vinay Prasad, who has a significant social media profile, has taken issue with precision medicine trial design in particular, especially relating to the lack of randomisation and replicability. This, in turn, has prompted criticism from advocates of personalised medicine, who suggest that flexibility is the new (and ethical) approach to meet patient needs, eschewing the rigid orthodoxies of the past.[8] Here we see some of the disputes about the promise of personalised cancer medicine laid bare as the valuation practices of trials are openly contested in professional and public forums.

We can situate the emergence of these trials and debates about their efficacy as part of the wider bioeconomy of promissory capitalism, where disease-free futures are continually re-envisaged (Cooper 2008; Michael 2017b). Expectations about personal and collective futures feature prominently in these regimes (Good et al. 1990; Novas 2006; Haase et al. 2015) as 'future-oriented discourses drive and shape innovation projects' (Borup et al. 2006: 285). Yet as Brown and de Graaf (2013) demonstrate, both hope and despair are key to trial arrangements in practice (see also Cooper 2008; Will and Moreira 2010; Cooper and Waldby 2014). The cultivation of low expectations among patients has also been shown to be a way in which clinicians manage the hype of contemporary biomedicine (Gardner et al. 2015), something we return to in Chapter 4.

Brown and de Graaf (2015) analysed the lived experiences of advanced cancer patients involved in phase 2 and phase 3 randomised control trials. Their research found that hope can be a means of managing the uncertainties associated with prognosis and treatment success. However, when negative eventualities and limited time horizons are introduced, patients engaged in 'bracketing off' the future, to limit reflection on the difficult realities that might lie ahead. These descriptions challenge conceptions of time as 'linear', with reflections on cancer necessarily encompassing an orientation towards the future in the present.

Montgomery's study of adaptive trials suggests that moving away from standardised approaches to 'predictable uncertainty' is premised on 'modes of knowledge production which claim to know the future' (2017b: 232). As trials speed up to deliver treatments to patients sooner, Montgomery argues that probabilistic logics are replacing promissory logics on which standard randomised trial designs are based. Here, adaptive trials are oriented around negotiation of unknowns as part of ongoing experiments, creating moral value, not just commercial value, for a diversity of actors. Optimisation through adaptability and iteration becomes key here, maximising the best possible future for patients amid uncertainty. Montgomery notes that such benefit tends to be framed as collective rather than as one for individual patients. There is a need to explore the implications of these processes for patients as they go through these trials.

We know from other studies that what Lamprell et al. (2018) aptly call 'the road of trials and obstacles' places numerous demands on patients. In their study of cancer patients' experiences of BRAF mutation testing, targeted treatments and associated trials, they discuss how BRAF mutation testing might be offered as part of efforts to secure access to a trial, but this is not a straightforward process. As in the case of one patient in their study, delays can mean that the trial closes before the tissue samples are analysed, and patients can find themselves having to transfer to another hospital to participate in the trial. Patients also have to manage a host of side-effects from experimental treatments accessed via trials, sometimes becoming too ill to continue. For others, accessing the drug via a trial can prove to be a lifeline, although not without ongoing complications to be lived with while in remission, with other drugs prescribed to manage side-effects. This points to the importance of patients' hope, trust and vulnerability in crafting futures in cutting-edge cancer care, themes also in Brown et al.'s research on the imperative of hope and trust in clinical trials (Brown et al. 2015).

We find echoes of this across our research, captured in the extract below, taken from a joint interview with two breast cancer patients, Laura and Viv. Both had late-stage cancer diagnoses when they had young families and were now living with secondary breast cancers.

They got to know each other through their secondary cancers, which put them 'in a completely different place [to primary cancer patients]', as Laura explained. During the interview, they talked about the work they had done to find out about trials and their advocacy around access to drugs. Viv received a standard treatment drug to which she responded well, whereas Laura, after receiving various chemotherapies, got on to a trial of a targeted therapy which she takes in tablet form alongside Herceptin. Laura told us she had secured the 'last place' on the trial, at a point when she had 'failed on quite a few lines of chemotherapy so ... was running out of options and ... probably only had less than six months to live'. She continues:

[Laura] I remember we went away to [city overseas] as a family because I kind of thought 'this might be my last big holiday'. And my consultant ... when I came back I thought I'd be going on possibly my last line of chemotherapy but when I got back he'd contacted his friend in [another city] and he said 'there's a slot on this trial'.

[...]

[Laura] ... there's an international trials database and I'd been sending ... my consultant, links to ... I remember trials in France and Belgium. And I think most of them were immunotherapy trials – I didn't know that – but he said to me 'oh, I'm not sure about these, it's still pretty untested in breast cancer, the response rate is very low. I really don't advise ... you'd have to go and live in Belgium or France or wherever for a number of months, is that feasible?' So he wasn't keen. But to be fair to him, he obviously did contact the [cancer centre in another city] and there was one place left on this trial and I thought 'I've got nothing, absolutely nothing to lose.' But no, he knew nothing about my, you know, molecular profile at all. But within a fortnight my cough had gone, I felt I was, you know...

[Viv] It was quite miraculous, actually.

[Laura] It was, it was a really strong, very strong response. And after three cycles of the drug, I got scanned and the cancer in my lungs had been, you know, just obliterated and it stayed like that.

[Viv] The thing is, when you're dealing with that sort of possibility of a trial with the drugs that are coming through, you just think, you know, it should be advertised.

[Laura] It should be.

[Viv] It really should be.

[Laura] And it's just been pure chance, luck.

[…]

[Viv] You can understand why we do what we do because you just think you're given this second chance at life really, aren't you, by a drug and you just think 'OK, I might have two years or three years but I'm going to make that two years or three years matter within the whole scheme of breast cancer for women really.'

[…]

[Laura] What's frustrating for me though is the drug has been really successful. So … I know there were 11 of us on the trial. There's me and one other lady still on it after two years – I think sadly the other women have died. But I saw a poster presentation from the company and they said it's had a 67% response rate in this very early phase one trial.

[Viv] Which is amazing.

[Laura] Which for women who've been heavily pre-treated, it's a really good response rate.

[Laura] And they described it as being 'unprecedented' but for some reason they've not taken it forward to phase two. So when I tell my story at different places, I always have people coming up to me, saying 'what drug are you on, what trial is this?' And I have to say 'I'm really sorry but I'm kind of on it, I got the last place and they don't seem to be … at some point they'll take it forward but they don't seem in any…'

[Viv] … rush, yes. Right, let's just say 'you've got to do it, you've just got to do it!'

As this exchange suggests, participation can extend from negotiating individual access, in concert with clinicians, to include more concerted collective efforts to open up more trials and more access to trials for other patients. It also includes managing hopes and expectations for oneself and others as the research progresses, and when personal benefits and findings do or do not materialise. Patients can take an active role in challenging clinicians, not just in relation to their own treatments but trial design too. This has included challenges to the exclusion criteria for clinical trials, as in the example of a US physician, Dr Kelly Shannon, who has metastatic breast cancer and has campaigned with patient organisations METAvivor (established in 2009 to provide funds for research)[9] and METUP (formed in 2015 and drawing inspiration from the AIDS activists ACTUP)[10] to open up access to trials to patients who are not just what she describes as the 'healthiest of the dying'.[11] Patient representatives are also increasingly involved in trial-management processes via patient and public involvement advisory groups and panels. This is now a routinised feature of cancer research. But acting as a representative in complex adaptive trials and other kinds of studies such as whole genome sequencing initiatives, as discussed below, can involve detailed engagement with the complexities of genomic science as well as trial methodologies, project governance, engagement and ethics.

Yet as Llewellyn et al. argue, based on their research on patients with brain cancer, trials take place in the context of 'the contingent and improvised nature of care', where doubts and uncertainties can be overshadowed by 'an unduly optimistic and "can-do" attitude to management based around a technological imperative and medicine's mandate to extend lives' (Llewellyn et al. 2018: 413; see also Kaufman 2015). Focusing instead on the 'unsettling and wavering terrains of disease and care', they explore how patients navigate experimental treatments, necessitating detailed engagement with research, medical travel and NHS bureaucracy (Llewellyn et al. 2018: 411). This includes managing being excluded from participation in trials to access new therapies such as Avastin, a targeted chemotherapy (not available to one patient in their study due to his prior involvement in an immunotherapy trial abroad), as well as crowdfunding efforts to access drugs considered by the NHS to be of unproven benefit. These kinds of 'unimaginable dilemmas and hard-to-swallow paradoxes' are part of the terrain of targeted treatments for cancer (Llewellyn et al. 2018: 420).

It is also important to appreciate that patients who actively seek out trials do this from a range of backgrounds and perspectives, not always based on detailed engagement and knowledge. One oncologist gives an example of this:

> I've had a GP … being treated in another institution … phone because they've read on the internet about a clinical trial that was taking place that they've seen the inclusion criteria for that they want to be

included in. [But this goes] all the way through to people having absolutely no idea, you know, really what a clinical trial is, a clinical trial is being a guinea pig ... I've – somebody said it to me this week in fact ... bizarrely this person said it to me ... he said, 'Oh, I just want you to know ... that I'm quite happy to be a guinea pig.'

Adaptive trials of targeted treatments can make cancer patients partners in experimental healthcare, but the extent and type of their engagement in the processes of the trial, including its design, purpose and outcomes, varies considerably, as do their experiences of access and care. Trials might be based on optimising the future for patients as a whole, but individual patients are also heavily invested in extending their own future. Trials are complex, just like cancers and patients, which brings considerable negotiation and articulation work for patients and their practitioners, not just to enable access but to keep hope alive for patients in and around the trial, as we discuss further in Chapter 4.

Whole genome sequencing

Developments in large-scale genomic sequencing are another feature of clinical oncology and associated research. More genetic information is being collected about more kinds of cancers, often through research studies. Whole genome sequencing (WGS), in which the entire genome is sequenced rather than panels (or groups) of genes – an approach associated with molecular diagnostic tests (often proprietary) and targeted treatments – is an important aspect of these developments. As Nakagawa and Fujita comment,

Whole genome sequencing (WGS) approaches can be used to comprehensively explore all types of genomic alterations in cancer and help us to better understand the whole landscape of driver mutations and mutational signatures in cancer genomes and elucidate the functional or clinical implications of these unexplored genomic regions and mutational signatures. (2018: 513)

WGS has a profoundly exploratory logic, charting previously unknown territories of the genome to reveal its complexity (Martin 2018). As Brown and Michael (2003) note, innovative technologies often build upon past 'failures' while ignoring the possibility of their own failure. This pattern appears to be being replicated in the case of WGS: its role in transforming cancer care is being assured through major infrastructure developments in the NHS, and the lack of ensuing 'actionable results' is not being framed as problematic.

At this point, genomics meets biobanking, often incorporating other clinical datasets where patients have given consent for their data to be reused. Digital processes of analysis are crucial to handling these vast quantities of data, as are private–public partnerships to deliver the technology and interpretative power required. The creation of value from these datasets requires both the centralisation of data and its ultimate detachment from the state (Cool 2016), in a process through which populations become brands with bioeconomic potential (Tupasela 2017). The promise of a growing bioeconomy aligns with a vision of health services that deliver better care to more patients via 'benefit sharing' (Hayden 2007), for example, where companies offer medical innovations to the health service that provide the data at a preferential rate. Yet these benefits remain opaque and promissory, sometimes bewildering to patients and participants already caught up in 'surveillance capitalism' where rights to privacy are routinely signed away as part of ordinary consumption (Zuboff 2019), and where publicly funded health systems are struggling to pay for expensive medicines such as targeted cancer therapies. How the 'regularized, embodied work that members of the national population are expected to perform in their role as biobank participants' (Mitchell and Waldby 2010: 334) is to be recognised or rewarded in such contexts is radically unclear. The ethical complexities of this are compounded in cancer, where benefits may not be felt, futures compromised and legacies uncertain.

Tarkkala et al. explore some of these dynamics in their research on personalised medicine in Finland – 'an intensely state-driven and national endeavour' (2019: 143) – analysing detailed policy plans and institutional strategies for embedding personalised medicine in Finnish healthcare. This work spans 'business, from financing to marketing, resource and personnel management, scientific research, product development, consulting, and public governance and poli-cymaking ... experimenting with existing epistemic, professional, institutional, political, legal, administrative, and business orders' (Tarkkala et al. 2019: 143–4). Wealth creation is a central theme of these efforts, realised via intensified innovation, commercialisation and data-driven medicine, which they note builds on two decades of promise that can be traced to the development of deCode Genetics Ltd in Iceland (Fortun 2008; see also Rajan 2006).

The discourses that surround these ventures are highly promissory, focused on delivering benefits to the nation, as well as patients and individual participants, but often hedging the later possibilities against the complexities and risks of the processes and the need for new infrastructures to be developed. Institutions are constructed as slow or even resistant to change and the success of WGS is predicated on transforming laboratory services and professional cultures, echoing the democratising ethic of corporate actors such as 23andme (Prainsack 2017). As well as recruiting patients as active collaborators in its genesis and implementation, health systems too need to be made ready for personalised medicine as expressed in policy documents such as the following:

> Predicting which patients will benefit ahead of time, using information from an individual's cancer genome to improve overall outcomes and minimise toxicity and cost, is the clear path forward. To achieve these goals, health systems need to evolve from their current state, to a more personalised model of cancer care with targeted therapies, driven by more precise and genome-driven research and diagnostics. This is a central tenet of Precision Medicine. (Scottish Scientific Advisory Council 2019: 5)

Just as new institutional requirements to better manage interpretation and clinical decision making based on results emerge from these innovative, commercially oriented, data-intensive initiatives, so too do new arrangements for the professional training and ethics required to support data generation, curation and exploitation. Consent to participate in research and the management of so-called 'incidental' findings supplementary to a patient's cancer (typically in relation to genetic risk for inherited disease) are a particular focus of attention here, given the importance of widespread participation to the success of these ventures (Dheensa et al. 2018). But these are complex endeavours, marked by numerous misalignments between policy, strategy and practice, given the complexities and pressures of healthcare systems. In the UK, and the NHS in England within it, the 100,000 Genomes Project is an exemplar of the kinds of large national initiatives that are delivering WGS, which we discuss further in Chapter 5.

Conclusion

The promise of personalised or precision medicine for cancer is contested in medicine, science and beyond in the public sphere because of concerns about efficacy and cost in particular. As Interlandi (2016) argues, 'early attempts to tailor disease treatment to individuals based on their DNA have met with equivocal success, raising concerns about a push to scale up such efforts'. Tim Maughan, from the CRUK/MRC Oxford Institute for Radiation Oncology, notes that personalised medicine for cancer has thus far proven to be of limited clinical benefit, quoting a study which found that 'overall survival from 71 targeted cancer therapies approved by the FDA between 2002 and 2014 was only 2.1 months' (Fojo et al. 2014). He continues:

> The consequences of heterogeneity, clonal evolution and the influence of the host response are that simple genetic tests are much less accurate in predicting prognosis and treatment response than was expected based on the CML imatinib paradigm. Similarly, targeted drug therapies may show an initial response, but this is rapidly overtaken by tumour regrowth due to emergence of tumour clones often demonstrating multiple different mechanisms of resistance. Despite this, personalised cancer medicine, now enhanced by immunotherapy, is still projected as the existing paradigm, and supported by major cancer centres across the world, by pharmaceutical and diagnostic companies alike. *Researchers* in the field and especially pharmaceutical companies are acutely aware of the challenges, *but still clinicians, patients and their advocates pursue access to these targeted agents with enthusiasm.* (Maughan 2017: 15) [our emphasis]

Maughan captures the key dynamic of anticipation and concern that we find across the various developments in genomic medicine for cancer reviewed in this chapter and explored further in the chapters that follow. Personalised cancer medicine is replete with promissory claims and instances of optimism and hope. Yet these tropes and possibilities are fragile and contested, when they emerge in everyday encounters, collective action and in the more stylised pronouncements in policy and the media.

What we stress here, however, is that these activities need to be understood as part of, rather than auxiliary to, the innovative and experimental processes in personalised medicine for cancer.

Innovation and experimentation extend outwards from the dataset or the laboratory, the scientist or the entrepreneur, to the clinic and beyond, to the regulatory and public sphere, and in networks and relations with fellow cancer patients, families and friends. Across these settings, practitioners, patients and their families are doing emotional and articulation work (Star 1985) as they co-produce the meanings of novel genomic treatments, tests, research and relations, crafting their and others' futures as part of this process. Anticipation and moderation are part of navigating individual and collective futures and creating various kinds of value, from the big futures of bioeconomic growth for the nation to individual, more personal futures of feeling cared for and valued. Just as molecular diagnosis, targeted therapy and subtypes of cancer and cancer research and care are entwined, interactive and co-produced, so too are individual and collective futures. These experimental relations, processes and categories enrol increasing numbers of patients and practitioners not just in research or data collection but in new kinds of regulatory and funding arrangements, patient collectives and public engagement activities.

In what follows, we endeavour to explore these interactions and interweavings to give a detailed account of the kinds of value that various sorts of work create as genomics personalises cancer medicine. We explore the activities and narratives of patients, practitioners and family members that make genomic medicine valuable in policy and in practice but can be hidden or unacknowledged. Looking at the kinds of futures being crafted and how experimental and articulation work in personalised medicine for cancer is distributed and enacted across these settings, we go on to consider what happens when we begin to value it as a contribution to innovation, and how this might change how we share the benefits and risks of personalised cancer medicine now and in the future.

Notes

1 Precision Medicine Initiative, https://allofus.nih.gov/about/program-overview/precision-medicine-initiative-data-security-policy-principles-and-framework-overview (accessed 3 October 2019).

2 http://news.bbc.co.UK/1/hi/health/5063352.stm (accessed 20 June 2020).

3 'Research shows breast cancer recurrence halved', press release, Roche, 3 June 2005 https://www.scoop.co.nz/stories/GE0506/S00017.htm (accessed 20 June 2020).

4 The Institute of Cancer Research, *Improving access to innovative cancer drugs*, December 2018, p. 3, www.icr.ac.UK/drugaccess (accessed 20 June 2020).

5 www.itv.com/news/wales/2019-03-19/mum-who-lives-half-a-mile-over-welsh-border-denied-life-prolonging-cervical-cancer-drug/ (accessed 20 June 2019).

6 SHIVA was the first clinical trial of molecularly targeted drugs for the off-label treatment of heavily pretreated metastatic cancer, at the Institut Curie, France (see www.thelancet.com/journals/lanonc/article/PIIS1470-2045(15)00458-1/fulltext (accessed 20 June 2020)).

7 T. Cynober, 'SHIVA trial, France's big shot at precision medicine', 20 July 2017, https://labiotech.eu/features/shiva-trial-precision-medicine-cancer/ (accessed 20 June 2020).

8 See P. Goldberg, 'Vinay Prasad, oncologist and Twitter star, locked in debate over precision medicine', The Cancer Letter, 2018, https://cancerletter.com/articles/20180622_1/ (accessed 20 June 2020).

9 www.metavivor.org (accessed 20 June 2020).

10 http://metup.org (accessed 20 June 2020).

11 https://medivizor.com/blog/2018/04/05/patient-activist-and-researcher-dr-kelly-shanahan-part-3/ (accessed 20 June 2020).

2

Genomic techniques in standard care: gene-expression profiling in early-stage breast cancer

Breast cancer has long been a focus of research and innovation in genomic medicine, from one of the first targeted therapies, Herceptin, as discussed in Chapter 1, to testing for mutations in breast cancer susceptibility genes such as BRCA1 and BRCA2, which developed through the course of the 2000s. Research into the molecular biology and gene expression of breast cancer tumours has spurred the identification of a range of variants or subtypes of breast cancer according to their molecular make-up. In addition to the development of Herceptin for HER2 breast cancers, estrogen receptors were also identified as targets for drugs in women with breast cancer before the menopause who had what is known as hormone-sensitive breast cancer. Cancers were classified into a range of subtypes according to genomic and other tests in the ensuing period. Olopade et al. reported that

> individual cancers could be categorized, based on their gene signature, to at least five distinct subtypes: luminal A, luminal B, normal-like, HER2-like, and basal-like. Normal-like tumors resemble normal breast tissue, HER2-like are characterized by HER2 overexpression, luminal A and B are estrogen receptor positive, and basal-like are triple negative (estrogen receptor negative, progesterone receptor negative, and HER2 negative). (2008: 7991)

These developments were the outcome of considerable research investment by public bodies, charities and commercial companies. Cancer research has been enabled, in part, by strong traditions of community and advocacy among breast cancer patients focused on prevention, research and survivorship in particular (Nahuis and Boon 2011; Gabe et al. 2012). Together, breast cancer research and activism are considered to have made major inroads into tackling the disease. Many breast cancers are now highly treatable when detected early, and UK survival rates have doubled in the last four decades, bringing ten-year survival rates for women up to 78 per cent across England and Wales for those cancers diagnosed early (Cancer Research UK 2014).

Sequencing and microarray technologies arising from the human genome project have enabled gene-expression profiling within cancer medicine. This technique identifies which genes are being activated in a cell to give a global picture of cellular function.[1] Oncotype DX is a gene-expression test developed by a US-based company, Genomic Health. It aims to provide a personalised prediction for a subset of breast cancer patients for whom the benefit of chemotherapy after surgery is less clear. The test estimates the likelihood of recurrence and can thus aid decisions about chemotherapy (Bourret et al. 2011). As Dowsett and Dunbier note, Oncotype DX was one of several 'multigene expression profiles that aim[ed] to outdo traditional predictive and prognostic factors' in breast cancer diagnosis and treatment, developed to 'quantify the residual risk of … recurrence in patients with lymph node negative, estrogen receptor-positive tumors receiving tamoxifen' (2008: 8022).

Echoing ongoing discourses of optimistic and transformative futures associated with genomic medicine, Oncotype DX has been hailed by some commentators as a key tool to combat the over-treatment of patients via chemotherapy (Joh et al. 2011; Ali-Khan et al. 2015). This has been welcomed because of its potential benefits for individual patients and practitioners in deciding on whether to recommend chemotherapy to prevent the recurrence of cancer, despite its sometimes serious side-effects and the disruption this causes (Bell 2009). Reducing unnecessary chemotherapy could also save resources within the UK NHS (Loncaster et al. 2017), although use of this test is primarily to help define who, from a subset of patients, would benefit from chemotherapy.[2]

As we discussed in Chapter 1, gene-expression profiling tests such as Oncotype DX have also been part of a wider transformation in innovation and regulation. This has involved novel partnerships between commerce and healthcare, with tests utilising proprietary algorithms. It has also involved new regulatory arrangements and pressures, marked by complex negotiations in state-based health systems such as the UK's, involving multiple stakeholders from healthcare, industry and patient advocacy. As of 2018, the National Institute for Clinical Excellence recommends three such tests: Oncotype DX, EndoPredict and Prosigna, replacing its previous 2013 guidance which included MammaPrint (see below). These tests have been introduced into an already busy diagnostic and treatment nexus in the NHS, which is not only non-linear, but is also already populated with a range of information and expectations, to which additional molecular information adds another layer. This means that, although molecular testing might promise certainty, it brings additional kinds of uncertainties too, all of which have to be navigated by researchers, patients and clinicians in the clinic and beyond.

In this chapter we look at these processes more closely, exploring the ways in which Oncotype DX, as one tumour-profiling test, has been made valuable to the health service, practitioners and patients, including via patients' contributions to processes of regulatory and clinical decision making surrounding the test. We chose to focus on Oncotype DX after discussing our research with senior clinicians in our project advisory group, who pointed out that we ought to include an aspect of genomic medicine already embedded in the clinic alongside the other case studies we were developing on genomic medicine as part of a trial or research. As we discuss further in Chapter 7, we had been finding entry into the clinic to study ordinary care difficult because of the complexities of patient pathways, clinical arrangements and ethical and governance approvals. However, clinicians were keen to understand patient experience of the test and of genomics more broadly, and helpfully assisted in recruitment for this case study, as well as being willing to be interviewed themselves.

This chapter considers transformations in policies and practices surrounding Oncotype DX and what sort of work this involves for patients and practitioners. We draw on research from three settings: the (public) approval process for the 2018 reformulation of UK NICE guidance around tumour-profiling tests; online patient discussions about Oncotype DX (between 2015 and 2017); and interviews with 18 patients who had had the test, interviews with nine healthcare professionals (between 2017 and 2019) and six observations of consultations (2017). To gather the online data, we searched for the term 'Oncotype' on publicly accessible online forums, hosted by cancer charity websites, and analysed discussion about Oncotype DX among cancer patients therein (Ross et al. 2019).

As we shall see, bringing Oncotype DX into routine practice involved considerable ongoing negotiation around evidence of benefit to the NHS and to patients and practitioners, as its meanings and implications were negotiated across a range of policy, practice and personal contexts. We explore how patients and practitioners worked to give the test value in their practice and experiences across these contexts, and we consider ambivalence about, and at times rejection of, its value. This ambivalence was centred on how the test could amplify, not simply resolve, uncertainty in already unstable treatment pathways regarding the role of adjuvant chemotherapy in this group of patients. Investigating how policymakers and NHS providers framed the test, we also highlight its precarious innovation pathway, exploring how its value had to be renegotiated across policy, community and clinical contexts. Despite the common claim that personalised genomic medicine is mainstream for cancers such as breast cancer because of the long-standing use of targeted treatments facilitated by gene-expression tests, our case study of Oncotype DX suggests a more precarious and contingent story of genomic medicine in the mainstream.

Gene-expression profiling within the UK NHS: crafting genomic futures

Commercial molecular profiling tests for breast cancer have become established since the early 2000s (Bourret et al. 2011; Kohli-Laven et al. 2011). MammaPrint is a 70-gene cancer signature developed and commercialised by the Dutch company Agendia, and Oncotype DX, which analyses 21 genes, was developed by the US company Genomic Health. Oncotype DX remains one of the NICE-approved tests, as noted above.

Oncotype DX is available to early-stage breast cancer patients with estrogen receptor positive (ER+) and human epidermal growth factor receptor 2 negative (HER2–) breast cancer tumour tissue which has not spread to lymph nodes (LN–) where a clinician is unsure about whether they will benefit from chemotherapy to prevent recurrence. It is important to note that this patient group is quite specific – they are already at low risk of recurrence and Oncotype DX may be used to help determine whether adjuvant chemotherapy might be beneficial. There is variation in the prognoses for these cancers (Nagaraj and Ma 2013), and for some of these patients the risks of chemotherapy, including long-term side-effects, can outweigh any potential utility in reducing the possibility of recurrence. Oncotype DX testing is typically performed when widely adopted risk-assessment calculators which look at markers such as ER and HER2 (e.g. NHS Predict)[3] do not provide a sufficiently definitive recommendation with regard to treatment, placing these patients at what is described as an 'intermediate' or 'moderate' risk of cancer's return in the context of an overall low risk of such recurrence. In these cases, according to NICE guidelines, clinicians can offer Oncotype DX testing (the list price is £2,580 and the discounted cost to the NHS is commercially confidential).[4] This involves sending tumour tissue, taken at surgery, to a Genomic Health licensed laboratory in the United States for molecular profiling of the 21 genes it analyses. The Oncotype DX test generates a personalised prediction for cancer survival with endocrine treatment (such as tamoxifen) alone, and based on this, a quantitative assessment of chemotherapy benefit. This is represented as a numerical 'recurrence score' between 0 and 100, categorised into risk bands. Initially this involved 'low-risk', 'intermediate' and 'high-risk' groups, with those patients at higher and in some cases intermediate risk of recurrence recommended to undergo adjuvant chemotherapy, taking other factors such as age into account. These three categories were represented visually, with the patient's place on the scale and corresponding ten-year survival prognosis, with or without chemotherapy, highlighted on a graph. Recently, following the outcome of the TAILORx trial, results have been presented in two bands – low and high risk.[5]

When NICE first recommended Oncotype DX for NHS use in 2013 (NICE 2013), the announcement was widely welcomed in the UK media, prompting headlines such as 'New Breast Cancer Test Could Spare Women Chemotherapy' (Boseley 2013). Coverage positioned the test as an example of improvements to the health service which could arise from genomic techniques, with the chief executive of a national breast cancer charity declaring that its approval represented a 'step along the road towards personalised treatment' (Smyth 2013), echoing the big future promissory discourses that commonly accompany developments in cancer science. However, five years later, during a 2018 reformulation of NICE guidance for tumour-profiling tests, initial recommendations suggested that the test ought to be withdrawn because there was a lack of evidence of its benefit. The value of the test for the NHS had to be re-established by the manufacturer, practitioners and patients, as we now go on to discuss.

In January 2018 NICE released a public consultation document following an expert advisory group (EAG) review of available tumour-profiling technologies. Following their diagnostics assessment, including a systematic review of clinical evidence and updated economic analyses (Harnan et al. 2017), NICE's consultation document asserted that:

> There is not enough evidence to recommend the routine adoption of EndoPredict, MammaPrint, Oncotype DX Breast Recurrence Score, Prosigna and IHC4+C to guide adjuvant chemotherapy decisions … In particular, more evidence is needed to prove that these tests have a positive effect on patient outcomes. Their cost effectiveness compared with current practice is highly uncertain. (NICE 2018a)

NICE called for further research on the effect of these techniques on long-term patient outcomes and treatment decision making, when compared with established risk-calculation tools already used by clinicians to predict breast cancer recurrence, such as NHS Predict (NICE 2018a).

Though some stakeholders agreed with the EAG's initial assessment in the consultation document, their recommendation to withdraw Oncotype DX from NHS care was met with considerable criticism. Following a call for stakeholder responses to the public consultation document, NICE received 255 comments from a range of actors including NHS professionals, charities representing patients and manufacturers (NICE 2018c). For these critics, the withdrawal of gene-expression profiling from NHS care was at odds with the transformation of the health service envisaged within wider UK discourses of the genomic revolution; around 170 comments were received from healthcare professionals, the majority of whom reported that the test had transformed their practice. Objecting to the recommendation, they framed it as a retrograde step for the health service, with a minority citing concerns of a return to a one-size-fits-all approach to breast cancer treatment. For example, one professional wrote:

> Please do not reverse this recommendation which will have the knock on effect to reverse the progress made by NHS in breast cancer treatment in the UK and have a huge negative impact on so many ladies who do not need or deserve the terrible impact they will endure in both short and long-term from having chemotherapy. (NICE 2018c: Comment 78)

Alongside these appeals to the responsibilities of practitioners and the NHS to prevent the harm of unnecessary chemotherapy, others pointed to the certainty and 'relief' offered by the test, as in the excerpt below:

> Being able to request an Oncotype DX test for my breast patients where there is uncertain benefit has revolutionised my practice. It is difficult to put a price on the relief that a patient has when told that they do not need to have chemotherapy which is unlikely to help them. The more we can personalise treatment, the less wastage we shall have and be able to focus treatments on those who are likely to benefit. (NICE 2018c: Comment 1)

The responsibility of professionals and services to reduce waste and target resources at a time when services are already stretched was another common theme:

> In 2018 we cannot ignore the advances technology has given us and go back to the dark ages of giving chemotherapy to everyone 'just in case'. Our day units are too full, lets target our resources wisely and save patients from undergoing unnecessary treatments. (NICE 2018c: Comment 81)

These sentiments were also echoed by the charity Breast Cancer Now, which released a statement following the announcement of these draft recommendations:

> [It is] very disappointing that NICE has been unable to recommend any of these prognostic tools to help guide chemotherapy use on the NHS. In particular, this appears to be a backwards step for some patients ... for whom guidance published in 2013 previously recommended the use of Oncotype DX. With studies to assess their long-term impacts ongoing, prognostic tests like these are showing real potential to personalise breast cancer treatment and ensure all patients are

given the best chance of survival, while reducing overtreatment. (Breast Cancer Now 2018)

Here we see the deployment of a familiar trope of personalisation as future-oriented transformation by both patient advocates and practitioners, who also referenced collective responsibilities to support the NHS and not fall behind the rest of the world. Reducing toxic chemotherapy generates cost savings for the NHS and offers patients better health and emotional relief.

However, very few individual patients submitted comments. Only two out of 255 comments were from patients, both of whom were supportive of approval because it reduced the burden of chemotherapy, including this one:

> I was predicted a 70% survival rating by PREDICT (which you seem to think can take the place of genomic testing) as opposed to 98% by the Oncotype DX genomic test. I would have had to have chemo, the possible long-term drawbacks of which I do not think you have adequately taken into account in your documentation of the site. Not to mention the unquantifiable psychological effects of a relatively poor prognosis. (NICE 2018c: Comment 174)

This forms part of a broader pattern in NICE assessments of novel diagnostics and therapies, where evidence of benefit becomes a key terrain of dispute and epistemological activism (Keating and Cambrosio 2011) on the part of health economists and other policy experts, industry, practitioners and patients. A particular tension arises between the tendency of expert review groups to prioritise the evidence of overall benefit to the health service, while patient representatives and practitioners, sometimes in concert with industry, prioritise individual patient benefit, in this case the avoidance of the psychological and physical burden of unnecessary toxic therapies. Negotiations 'spill over' into the public sphere as part of the co-production of these kinds of NICE decisions (Moreira 2011: 1334), with the entitlements and 'moral worth' of patients forming part of the evidence that stakeholders mobilise alongside practitioners' and regulators' responsibilities to deliver value for money for the health service as a whole (Moreira 2011: 1338).

As Abraham (1995) and Davies and Abraham (2013) have shown, pharmaceutical companies influence regulatory processes affecting their products, including via funding clinical trials and working with regulators to speed up the approvals process. However, research has also shown that NICE committee members can be particularly sceptical about industry claims and those of patients who are seen as having conflicts of interest (Brown et al. 2016). The gene-profiling industry therefore adopted a muted tone in their submissions to the NICE committee, deploying a range of evidence of benefits and criticising the EAG for insufficient engagement with international study groups and trials.

However, it was the prospect of evidence from one trial that was particularly important in the advocacy work around Oncotype DX. Around thirty responses to the initial NICE report noted that the results of the Trial Assigning Individualised Options for Treatment (TAILORx) trial, a National Cancer Institute (US) sponsored large-scale prospective trial assessing the benefit of chemotherapy for those receiving 'intermediate' Oncotype DX scores, were shortly to be released, stressing the importance of this evidence to the process. In response, the Diagnostics Advisory Committee paused the development of their reformulated guidelines to conduct further analyses incorporating the trial results.

The TAILORx results were widely welcomed because they demonstrated that Oncotype DX offered more precise predictions, identifying the 70 per cent of women who would not benefit from chemotherapy (Sparano et al. 2018). The trial also found no need to use an intermediate score, as women in this category could be considered low risk and avoid chemotherapy. These results were reported with much fanfare in the UK media. When reporting on the technique and the TAILORx study, many news articles adopted terminology including 'life changing', 'ground breaking' (Matthews-King 2018) and a 'breakthrough' (Gallagher 2018). Headlines included 'Most Women with Early Stage Breast Cancer Can Avoid Toxic Chemotherapy' (*The Independent*) and 'Breast Cancer Study Set to Free Women from Chemotherapy' (*Financial Times*). Stories featuring personal testimonies included that of the *Guardian* journalist Joanna Moorhead, who recounted her own experience of Oncotype DX in the wake of the results of the TAILORx study, describing the technique as 'revolutionising' cancer treatment (Moorhead 2018).

These positive trial results, together with the arguments presented by contributors to the consultations, shaped NICE guidance, released in December 2018. During its final meeting, the NICE Diagnostics Advisory Committee reported scepticism about the applicability of TAILORx results to the UK. Many of those who avoided chemotherapy in this study would not have been routinely offered it in a UK setting, demonstrating that even so called 'gold standard' evidence is not always translatable to other health systems, affording clinicians, patients and regulators flexibility in interpretation and practice (NICE 2018b: section 5.6). Nonetheless, NICE retracted the earlier recommendation to withdraw support for Oncotype DX. The committee also recommended the adoption of Endopredict and Prosigna for use with ER+, HER2– and LN– early breast cancer patients in NHS settings, where certain criteria are met, including whether other validated tools such as NHS Predict had already suggested an intermediate risk, and that information would help patients to choose whether or not to have chemotherapy (NICE 2018b). In Moreira's study of dementia drug regulation, hybrid interactions between practitioners, patients and industry created the conditions for NICE to resolve disputes with pragmatic reasoning, balancing rules with individual cases, rendering the decision 'socially robust' rather than technocratic (Moreira 2011: 1340). We find similar processes in this case, as the regulator navigated a range of different types of evidence and advocacy around the value of the test for the NHS, practitioners and patients, recommending limited use of the test in conditions of uncertainty if the patient, together with their practitioner, would find this helpful.

In these processes of regulatory decision making we can see the articulation of value to patients and to the NHS being asserted and anticipated as an outcome of regulatory approval. The value to patients was articulated in evidence to the regulator, but this was largely second-hand rather than first-hand, via clinicians and patient advocates/representatives. The main form of value being asserted was the avoidance of unnecessary and expensive chemotherapy, something which was presented as mutually beneficial for patients and the NHS. Patients were also framed as deriving personal value from the test, which offered relief and prevented toxic side-effects when they could avoid chemotherapy with more certainty. The NHS was presented as deriving efficiency gains and financial benefits from these outcomes. The value of being 'future-oriented', not being backward or overtaken by other countries, was also asserted through these processes. Oncotype DX became totemic of the future of personalised medicine, generating a sense of shared commitment to its realisation (Jerolmack and Tavory 2014). Reducing suffering, saving money for the NHS and paving the way for further advances combined national and personal goals and benefits. For patients and practitioners, gene-expression profiling offered certainty and reassurance that they could avoid chemotherapy, resolving lingering uncertainties produced by other algorithms such as NHS Predict. For the NHS, the technology offered greater certainty by reducing wastage, and for policymakers and industry it made the future of personalised medicine less uncertain as the test became an option within standard care pathways.

However, when we turn to practitioners' and patients' accounts of engagement with Oncotype DX, we find it is associated with more complex and contingent value than the three kinds of value (personal value, value to the NHS, totemic value) discussed above. As in Hedgecoe's work on Herceptin (2005), the 'messy realities' of bringing Oncotype DX into treatment decision making meant that its value was contextually negotiated in practice. It was sometimes experienced as particularly valuable and unique, including because it is a novel commercial test, where tissue is processed in a US laboratory rather than an in-house hospital laboratory. On the other hand, it could also be experienced as unremarkable or lacking in special value, as just one of a raft of tests brought into decision making, and sometimes as lacking any additional value where its clinical utility was considered uncertain. All experiences involved patients and practitioners in particular kinds of emotional or articulation work (Star 1985), drawing on social and cultural capital to make meaning from the test in the here and now as well as for service and patient futures. This happened in the clinic and beyond in online breast cancer patient communities, as we now go on to examine.

Integrating genomic tumour profiling in practice

According to NICE guidelines, NHS clinicians are advised to administer gene-expression profiling in HER2+, ER– and LN– early-stage breast cancer where there is uncertainty around whether to recommend adjuvant chemotherapy to prevent recurrence, and where established tools such as NHS Predict are unable to offer a clear recommendation. This frames the test as a solution to such uncertainty. Yet as with many such tests, practitioners' experiences suggest that Oncotype DX is a means of managing rather than simply resolving uncertainty.

We interviewed nine practitioners involved with Oncotype DX in their practice, including one clinical nurse specialist, seven oncologists and one pathologist. We also carried out six observations of consultations where discussion of the Oncotype DX score took place, and where decisions were made regarding the benefit of adjuvant chemotherapy.

As practitioners in our study frequently pointed out, opting into or out of chemotherapy involves careful consideration of a patient's personal and social circumstances and clinical factors, where non-genomic quantified risk prediction through NHS Predict remains paramount in determining whether to offer gene-expression profiling. As in other fields, clinicians exercised their professional autonomy, non-routine working and tacit knowledge to work flexibly within NICE guidelines (Timmermans 2005; McDonald et al. 2006) when it came to Oncotype DX. Practitioners told us that decisions about Oncotype DX testing were not just based on the patient's cancer but included consideration of co-morbidities and individual patient characteristics, and in the words of one oncologist, their 'scope to benefit'. This flexibility is anticipated in the guidelines which require that 'information provided by the test would help them choose, with their clinician, whether or not to have adjuvant chemotherapy taking into account their preference'.[6]

We can illustrate how clinicians flexibly embed gene profiling in practice in collaboration with their patients through the account of one oncologist who reflected on their experience of treating a patient who had been resistant to undergoing chemotherapy because of the impact on their occupation. The oncologist had already determined that because the cancer was low grade, chemotherapy would not be a good option, and the Oncotype DX test simply confirmed this decision. As they stated, the test played a role in solidifying treatment recommendations that would already have been made: 'we feel really reassured that we're not doing the wrong thing. So that was really helpful for [the patient], but did it change our management? I don't know that it did.' As another oncologist attested, 'Quite frequently, it gives the result that you fully expected … It's more often that it's simply confirmed the view that we thought was more likely.' Similarly, during an observation of a consultation where the patient was categorised as 'high-risk' following Oncotype DX testing, the clinician confirmed that the patient would benefit from chemotherapy, a decision that they imply they would have reached regardless of the test:

> Speaking to the patient and her husband, the clinician explained that an additional test was required [didn't say why this was the case], which is called Oncotype DX, that tests a number of genes, '21 genes to be precise and based on this score, patients are categorised into 3 groups: "low risk", which is "good cancer", "intermediate' group, and the group with high risk of recurrence in 10 years.' The clinician confirmed that the patient is in the high risk group to which the patient's husband replied, 'yes, because it's 44%.' Based on this, the clinician went on to say 'I would have recommended chemotherapy anyway even without gene testing results.'

According to these accounts the value of the test was as a confirmatory device, reassuring patients and according with decisions reached using other clinical tools and judgements. In other consultations, however, and particularly for patients 'at the margins' with this lower-risk cancer, the Oncotype DX result was a means of providing further, and more precise, information which aided the decision about chemotherapy, as the extract below highlights:

> The consultant explained what the NHS Predict tool is and they went through each section together thoroughly. Because the patient is 'so young' [40 years old] the consultant predicted a good prognosis. They added that without the Oncotype test result [i.e. with just the NHS Predict result], it might have appeared that the patient doesn't need chemotherapy but with this result it shows the benefit – explaining they are 'trying to put different bits of information together'. The husband said 'given the cost of chemo', the benefit seems so small. The consultant said NHS Predict gives you 'a rough average' but because breast cancer is a big group of disease[s], this is 'where Oncotype comes in'.

The test was also used as a means of reassuring the patient's husband that chemotherapy would be beneficial given their concerns regarding efforts to balance the benefit and burden of chemotherapy. We see consultant, patient and relatives acting together to reach decisions, taking responsibility for obtaining specific information as part of this process.

This is also captured in a further observation with the same consultant:

> And then [consultant oncologist] gave an overview of the patient's cancer that it's common cancer and early grade (Grade 2 she said), 21 mm with clear margin, and ER+ & HER2–. [Consultant oncologist] then explained that breast cancer is a very big family of cancer [exactly same wording she used in the previous consultation I observed]. [Consultant oncologist] explained, by drawing a diagram on a sheet of A4 paper ('it's easier with a picture, isn't it?' the consultant said) – while explaining two subtypes of breast cancer which are estrogen receptor positive and negative, she wrote down ER+ and ER– on the sheet and then each ER+ and ER– is branched out by lymph node status i.e. positive and negative – I couldn't quite see from where I was sitting but I think they wrote down LN+ and LN– on the sheet. 'This is when Oncotype test comes in', [consultant oncologist] said – this looks at LN– within ER+ [categories] … 'on surface this cancer might look good but Oncotype might tell us otherwise' [this explanation is also very similar to what was said to another patient in consultation].

Here we see Oncotype DX being presented as providing certainty to resolve previous doubts around whether to proceed to chemotherapy, or even revealing more harmful cancers that might initially 'look good' on the surface, in the context of such a wide and varied 'family' of diseases. The test was valued by some clinicians because they felt it assisted patients who were finding decision making difficult. This is visible in the following extracts, from a discussion with a consultant following a clinical consultation and a separate interview:

> The consultation finished and the couple left the room to have a blood test done. Before I left, I asked the consultant if Oncotype DX is a useful tool and they said yes, as it helped the patient to change her mind or make up her mind.

> Patients often find it quite useful because it's difficult for them to make these decisions, so in a way having the test to tell you whether you should or shouldn't have chemotherapy takes the difficulty away from you and you just do what the test says. I think that's why a lot of patients quite like them.

In other situations, and for some other clinicians, the test was less useful. A clinical nurse specialist working with the technique noted that the test could not always offer certainty or eliminate the 'grey areas' experienced by patients and clinicians; nevertheless it was valuable because it was 'making them smaller'. After ordering gene-expression profiling many times, one clinician had almost stopped using the tool, now largely reverting to their prior practices of clinical judgement to make personalised decisions about chemotherapy treatment:

> The first year we did about eighty [patients] I think ... I don't know how many ... so what that showed to me was that almost nobody should get chemo ... they were all lower intermediate. So actually using it has been an education, because it reaffirms to me that I think almost nobody who has node negative breast cancer should get chemo. And now I think I've got enough data to feel confident about that, and that's why I think we don't need to get Oncotype to do that. So now I've kind of almost stopped using it ... because it's reaffirmed to me the UK backbone that was there all along, which was actually giving cytotoxic therapy to node negative hormone sensitive breast cancer, is almost always the wrong thing to do ... now how do you pick out the three or four women out of a hundred? Well maybe you can't, but how much benefit do those people get? In absolute terms not that much. And does Oncotype pick them out? We don't know because in the high risk group it was never randomised. TAILOR X assumed that the low risk group didn't need it, and assumed that the high risk did need it.

The oncologist above began using the test once it was recommended for funding, but found, over time, that their prior clinical experience and the decisions made were reinforced, not challenged, by Oncotype DX results, attenuating its value in practice. Nonetheless, the big future promises of personalised medicine remained, as they went on to say: 'I'm sure one day the computer will beat the human at chess, but I don't think Oncotype's the thing that's going to do it.'

We see, then, in common with other genetic tests as described by Latimer et al. (2006: 621), that Oncotype DX was just one of many resources involved in cancer diagnosis and prognosis, with the relationship between clinical judgement and laboratory testing complex, and by no means unilinear. This could include enacting professional responsibility to make judgements without tests that were perceived to be unnecessary, and questioning whether this test is an efficient use of limited resources, as the following oncologist describes:

> I suspect it's fulfilling its promise but at the downside of maybe quite a lot of tests are being done, that may not be, you know, for example, in patients that maybe, like you wouldn't really be giving chemotherapy to, but then you do it because they're eligible and it's low and you still don't give them chemo ... I just have slight concerns about how many, kind of, how accurately we're using them, you know, by throwing it around a lot. Some of them were hitting the mark, some of them are, are not. And just based on, kind of, how expensive it is and how bankrupt the health service is...

These more equivocal accounts of gene profiling strike a different tone to the optimism and anticipation reported in the UK media about Oncotype DX transforming practice, after the TAILORx trial and NICE consultation of 2018. They form a kind of 'backstage ambivalence' that enabled clinicians to embed the technique in practice, using it as part of a package of support, confirmation of diagnosis and prognosis, and management of patients' circumstances and expectations; yet a moderated frontstage commitment to such technologies can be maintained, as the oncologist quoted above went on to say:

> These sort of technologies are the future, they're not going to go away. Definitely they're going to stay ... but there may be a limit to how much predictive information you can get just from the cancer. Because the entirety of what's going to happen in that patient's next ten years is not just encoded in the cancer.

Being flexible also included situations where oncologists chose not to perform the test. For example, one oncologist described how they had chosen not to offer the test to one eligible patient because they did not consider it necessary:

> I had someone recently who was quite a young patient ... she had a grade three cancer and it was ... only moderately ER positive and so technically we could have done Oncotype on her. But I prejudged it that there was really minimal likelihood that it would come back with a low score and therefore didn't do it, just went ahead and gave chemo. I think doing the test almost certainly would have been a waste of the health service's money, because there's such a minuscule chance of it coming back low.

The potential delay that Oncotype DX testing could introduce to treatment pathways, with results taking around two weeks following shipment of the sample to the US-based laboratory, was also a source of concern.

All of this meant that there was considerable variation in the extent to which the clinicians we interviewed used the test, with some having used it on fewer than ten occasions. As suggested above, cost and patient care may have played a role here, but clinicians were also sceptical about the commercial interests behind the test, and the involvement of the manufacturer in the evidence base that supported its adoption in standard practice, echoing Hedgecoe's (2005) findings about Herceptin use being limited due to cost considerations.

The low usage among some clinicians interviewed was also associated with their high satisfaction with the standard tools and techniques used to estimate recurrence and chemotherapy benefit within the UK. UK pathology practice was framed as more comprehensive than in the US, where Oncotype DX was developed and trialled. Clinicians described feeling confident in the pathology reports used in the UK (these include markers not used in the US), and doubted the additional value provided by gene-expression profiling. One oncologist praised the pathologists they worked with in their practice, noting that they were very 'accurate' and provide a 'good rock' for clinical decisions. This was echoed by another, who contrasted pathology in the UK with the US:

> [Oncotype DX] adds a lot less to UK practice than it might have been expected to add to US practice ... and that's important when, in trying to understand the implications and trials like TAILORx which ... were predominantly run in the US ... which in our opinion probably has been, overtreating people for quite a long time with chemotherapy in, in groups of patients that we would have used existing prognostic parameters to identify.

These accounts differ from the clinical practitioner contributions to the NICE consultation, which emphasised the value of Oncotype DX to the NHS as a means of reducing waste and making cost savings, and instead echo some of the scepticism about over-interpretation of TAILORx trial results as expressed in the committee deliberations that followed. Here, Oncotype DX is framed as an unnecessary cost in a system that is already able to deliver high levels of prognostic precision, and we see these clinicians rearticulating arguments about value to the NHS as a reason *not* to use the test.

Alongside these multiple rearticulations of value and responsibilities with respect to clinical decision making, guiding patients and being cost-conscious, elsewhere clinicians intimated that Oncotype DX and other gene-expression profiling technologies were part of the future of the NHS, as evidenced in our examples. The promise of genomic medicine reflected in the NICE consultation and responses to TAILORx results was recapitulated in even otherwise ambivalent accounts. This hopeful view for the longer-term future of genomic cancer medicine was also held by one oncologist who had been particularly sceptical about the added value provided by Oncotype DX testing. The fact that this was an 'old' technology impacted their view of genomic profiling in breast cancer; however, they maintained a view that in the future there is the possibility of 'major impacts':

> You see Oncotype DX is old, whereas some of, some of the lung cancer mark[er], receptors are really quite, they are making a difference. So in a way Oncotype is old news, and I think there are other cancers, and it's not my expertise, but there are other cancers where there are markers or things that can be, that do definitely define pathways and outcomes and information regards in prognosis. So I think it will impact actually. I think maybe breast cancer will impact less than some others. But other cancers, definitely there may be some major impacts.

These clinicians did not describe gene-expression profiling for breast cancer – presented in some accounts as a 'poster child' for the movement of genomic techniques from bench to bedside – as revolutionary or transformative to their practice; in fact, many noted instead their satisfaction with long-established procedures. But in other respects, they mirrored public and policy contributions which positioned techniques such as gene-expression profiling as totemic of 'the future' of cancer care, maintaining anticipation while managing uncertainties in present practice.

This representation of the future of genomic medicine as on the cusp, but not quite attained, is a familiar trope that can be found in public discourse since the sequencing of the human genome almost twenty years ago. While this kind of 'genohype' has been a concern for stakeholders, including policymakers as they attempt to reconcile it with the pressures of a constrained health service, such expectations for genomic medicine have also been recognised as a stimulus and as necessary to drive clinical change (Samuel and Farsides 2017). Ambivalence and flexibility in the use of gene profiling in practice functions alongside anticipation as part of these processes of change. For practitioners, flexibility and ambivalence about the value of the test was part of managing uncertainties in the clinic while maintaining optimism about improved services and prospects for patients in the future. Clinicians' various renderings of the test as totemic of the future, confirmatory, provisional, incremental, and even at times obsolete, do not necessarily diminish but rather repurpose its value as an additional tool and another step along the way in improving cancer care. These accounts and activities are part of the articulation work through which they exercised professional responsibilities to their patients and the service as a whole.

Treatment decision making for early-stage breast cancer: patient accounts of Oncotype DX

In addition to the observations of consultations already discussed above, we also interviewed 19 breast cancer patients with experience of Oncotype DX (the majority of whom had the test as part of NHS care) and analysed 132 discussion threads on Oncotype DX from a total of seven online cancer patient forums. In this case study, patients' narratives had a different form and emphasis than the clinicians' interview accounts or their contributions to public consultations about the test. As with our other case studies, personalised medicine and genomic tests were but one part of patients' stories of cancer diagnosis and treatment, which encompassed a range of experiences of tests, treatments, research and care. This was the case with Oncotype DX too. Patients, on the whole, did not make a detailed case for or against the technology, nor did they articulate an elaborate vision for personalised medicine and its place within the NHS. Instead they narrated intricate stories of managing uncertainty, interpreting information, making choices, coping with feelings of hope and disappointment, pain and frailty and living through cancer with families and friends. Oncotype DX, like other tests, featured in these accounts sometimes as a key actor (for example, in online forum discussions about what to do after surgery or when detailing its role in decision making), but it was more typically surrounded by a multiplicity of narratives about treatment, care and research.

Within this context, Oncotype DX was loosely framed as an advance by most patients who had experienced the test, for example when they compared their experiences with the care received by friends and relatives, particularly because the test was costly and sometimes because it was performed in the US. Patients faintly echoed some of the promissory discourses of personalisation that we have identified in media and policy accounts. One patient, Bethany, who described the technique as 'state of the art', told us she worked in an environment where any change to her appearance would be noticed and commented upon, so she desperately wanted to avoid chemotherapy, articulating her responsibility to remain active and competent in the workforce despite her cancer. However, because the test was seen by her as authoritative, due to its being more 'advanced' than existing techniques, she conceded that should the result indicate she was at a high risk, the responsible thing to do would be to proceed to chemotherapy: 'I thought if a sort of state-of-the-art test is saying that's what I need then of course, it might be unpleasant but of course I'll go through that, you know, I'll have chemotherapy.' The scientific basis of the test was also a feature of its promise, as described by another patient, Julie: 'I was very pleased when I heard how the test worked because I thought "right, that's fine because that makes it much more specific and that will make me feel I'm not making a hunch decision, I'm making a decision based on actual science, actually related to me"'.

The advanced nature of the test was also referenced in online forums where some participants contrasted Oncotype DX with more widely used tools such as NHS Predict, positioning these as 'low-tech' when compared with gene-expression profiling. One user pointed to a dissatisfaction with established recurrence-risk estimation tools such as NHS Predict, which she noted 'I can access myself' (breast cancer charity forum). For these women Oncotype DX 'is a lot more personal and specific than the original %s' (cancer charity breast cancer forum), because 'generalised tools could be very wrong' (breast cancer charity forum).

For patients such as this, Oncotype DX testing is a way to enact their responsibility to choose wisely, as it was considered to offer more certainty than established tools predicting risk. Patient accounts have much more congruence with the kinds of value articulated in the consultation responses discussed above, particularly in terms of aiding difficult decisions and offering personal relief and reassurance. This was the case for interviewees such as Alice. Like others we spoke to, she described a very 'quick' experience of her breast cancer diagnosis and treatment with a clear set of procedures to engage with, until the possibility of chemotherapy was raised by her clinician. Following Alice's surgery, it was found that one of her lymph nodes was 'slightly affected' by the breast cancer, and the benefit/risk measure in her particular case for proceeding to chemotherapy was unclear. As Alice described, it was 'touch and go' from both her perspective and that of her oncologist, because the spread was 'such a small amount'. Alice wanted to avoid chemotherapy due to her wish to return to 'normal', and an understanding of the treatment as potentially 'worse than the cancer itself'. She described Oncotype DX as a 'perfect fit for what I wanted to understand about … chemo', and positioned the test as providing certainty in the context of complex treatment decisions:

> I need certainty. I said, right, I'll pay for this test if necessary, to make me make the right decision (laughing) … if I needed chemo, then I would just have to knuckle down and get it done … I just needed some certainty, as to whether I needed it or not.

Here Alice articulates her desire for certainty, and assumed responsibility for obtaining the test by paying for it herself if necessary. She was intending to act on the results, accepting chemotherapy if it was recommended, just to 'get it done'. Alice's feelings about Oncotype DX were echoed by Julie, who was very keen to avoid chemotherapy due to her concerns about her immunity being compromised during treatment; but she also felt that the treatment would be unavoidable if the test results predicted a high risk of recurrence. She described the information provided by the test as a 'crystal ball'.

These framings were also observed in online forum discussions. When users asked for information about the test, Oncotype DX was presented positively by some because, in the words of two respondents, it 'took the guesswork out of whether you should have chemo' and meant the patient would 'know whether you need chemo or not', offering one kind of certainty in an uncertain future. Collectively, patients on these forums encouraged and supported each other to take on the responsibility of accessing and acting upon Oncotype DX results. Oncotype DX was also praised by some as a means to aid chemotherapy decisions because of the way in which results are displayed as a single score representing recurrence risk and potential benefit from chemotherapy. Patients who had until that point experienced uncertain and shifting diagnostic pathways were particularly enthusiastic about this kind of scoring system. Oncotype DX testing was therefore valued by patients who told us they had found the uncertainties and 'false horizons' of diagnosis and treatment difficult. This was especially the case for those patients who had not initially anticipated having to consider chemotherapy, as it was not raised as a possibility until pathology results were obtained following surgery. For these patients, Oncotype DX results offered welcome guidance for an unexpected and unwelcome decision. Lillian, for example, told us of her experience of researching Oncotype DX online after her clinical nurse specialist (CNS) rang her to inform her about the test. Until this point, Lillian, an office worker in her early sixties, thought her cancer was a mucinous breast cancer, which is a rare cancer, but when she found out this wasn't the case, for her, 'it was kind of a sense of relief almost (laughs) … Because I thought, well, they're more used to treating a more common cancer.' Lillian found the CNS and online chatrooms were particularly useful in offering reassurance that the test was valuable for guiding treatment decisions. Of her Oncotype DX result, Lillian explained:

> I think I could see things in black and white a bit more clearly. So you can be told your grade or your stage of your tumour, but to be able to know a bit more about likely recurrence and a bit more about prognosis and things like that, for me … it all came together and made it so much more understandable somehow.

For Lillian, being a 'good patient' involved taking on the mantle of responsibility to research and consider options, to understand and make sense of results and to choose wisely when it came to treatment possibilities. This also encouraged Lillian to take part in the 100,000 Genomes Project (discussed in Chapter 5).

In some cases, where participants were placed in the low recurrence risk category, the test also enabled them confidently to avoid chemotherapy. Susan, whose daughter also had breast cancer at a similar time, explained that the Oncotype DX result 'reinforced' her preference for rejecting chemotherapy. Seeing her daughter struggling with chemotherapy, 'it was only because [of the] Oncotype result' that she could avoid the temptation of 'belt and braces sort of way of doing'. Bethany, meanwhile, described the test as allowing her to feel more 'confident' that it was not irresponsible to forego the treatment. The test results were also welcomed by some patients who were considered to be at a higher risk of recurrence and who might therefore benefit from chemotherapy to reduce that risk. Lois, who had her cancer detected at a three-yearly breast screening, described the meaning of the Oncotype test as 'a second opinion' which allowed her to avoid chemotherapy:

> [They said] 'we could just give you chemo or there is this test available, the Oncotype test' so immediately we said 'yes please, if we could get that'. And fortunately three weeks later it came back to say it was reading 6 so I was clear of needing any chemo so that was a great, a great day.

In other respects, however, certainty was not always provided by a straightforward reading of the test results, even when these were clearly at one or the other end of the spectrum, as the following example illustrates. Zoe, a medical professional, described her sense that there was a 'right' choice to be made about chemotherapy when she told us about her experience of the Oncotype DX. Using NHS Predict her cancer had been designated as at low risk of recurrence, but her oncologist voiced uncertainty about this designation because the cancer was high grade. Oncotype DX testing was recommended and Zoe started reading academic journal articles about the test, including the recent results of the TAILORx study. However, Zoe did not feel secure in rejecting chemotherapy when her Oncotype results came back with a low score of 7, and she deferred to her oncologist following the result, to further confirm that she was making the 'right choice'. Without Oncotype DX testing, she explained, because her cancer was high grade it would have been a 'constant worry' whether not going for chemotherapy was the 'right thing to do'. But it took work on the part of Zoe and her consultant to interpret the results of the test together in such a way as to achieve her sought-after certainty.

As clinicians emphasised, the interpretation of results was highly contextual. This is illustrated in the extract from fieldnotes below, in which an intermediate result is discussed:

And then [consultant oncologist] brought up Oncotype test results on the screen saying 'Graph is very useful'. [Consultant oncologist] said 'your score is 30 so it's intermediate risk'. The consultant said, 'hormone therapy will be beneficial but the difficult decision is about chemo'. The consultant asked the patient to guess where they 'belong' – the patient answered 'middle group' with a burst of laughter. The consultant showed the graph on the screen again and compared the risk of recurrence when the patient has hormone therapy (14%) vs. when she has both chemo & hormone therapy (7%). In order to emphasise the difference, the consultant used her fingers to measure the gap. The patient replied by saying, 'noticeable benefit'.

This is when the consultant brought up the patient's heart failure and the patient asked how much chemo will affect her heart condition. [Consultant oncologist] explained that any chemo drugs that might affect the patient's heart won't be allowed to [be] prescribe[d] and also because of the patient's history of pneumonia and kidney stone, alternative chemo drug called taxol will be recommended and the patient will be monitored very carefully. It's 'a diluted form' and will be administrated weekly so it's 'not too bad'. [consultant oncologist] then went on to explain the side effects including hair loss (the patient laughed), infection, and weight gain – the patient laughed again at this and turned to her mother and joked 'it will look really nice mom'. The consultant said they appreciated that the patient's heart condition is 'a significant setback' given that she always has reservation for chemo under any circumstance. The patient said she is 'between a rock and a hard place' but she has always been 'an unlucky person.'

Then the conversation shifted to talk about the patient's care responsibility. The patient's adult son is living with her and her husband and he has severe disability. The patient was concerned about her husband who is in his late 60s, which mean[t] he won't be able to look after their son on his own so she was wondering whether she will be well enough to continue to help out while receiving chemotherapy. The patient said this is the reason why 'this is difficult decision to make'. The consultant said 'I am glad you said this' and it's important to know what kind of 'limited reserve' the patient has. The patient said, 'I am a mess'. The consultant said it's possible to suspend chemo depending on the patient's general health and the patient replied 'it's reassuring to know' and suggested that she might 'try and see'. The consultant explained again that they will recommend the chemo that is for frail patients or patients with existing health issues and suggested that the patient can read information leaflet that will be given to her and have a think about it. The patient said she is happy about this arrangement so she could have a discussion with her family. They went on to talk a bit more about other side effects. The patient's mother asked if there is any alternative to chemo. The consultant reiterated the value of Oncotype test – there are some benefits of different treatment options but Oncotype test 'teases out' the benefits.

For this patient and her family, the intermediate test presented a 'difficult decision' given her health and caring responsibilities, and required careful negotiation over the kind of chemotherapy that she could manage. Together with the consultant and her mother, she worked to articulate and balance her various responsibilities to be well and to care for herself and her family, making the Oncotype DX result, and more specifically the intermediate result, a valuable tool for navigating her particular circumstances. The uncertainty of the intermediate result was productive, creating a space for consideration of this patient's unique circumstances, and facilitating her and her family's involvement in treatment decision making (see also Brown and de Graaf 2013; Swallow 2019).

As with the clinicians we interviewed, some patients also took other factors into account when making their decisions, rather than following the recommendations of their test result alone. Supported by her oncologist, one patient 'in the grey area' decided to go ahead with chemotherapy:

> so, my understanding anyway was that it's a low risk cancer but obviously the score on the Oncotype having been fed into that system … I was in the grey area as to, as to whether or not I would need [chemotherapy]. But in my head I'd already decided that it was inevitable.

Another woman with a low risk of recurrence score, writing on a breast cancer forum, noted that because of her young age and her experience of her father's death from bone cancer she would proceed with chemotherapy, despite her Oncotype DX result suggesting a low risk of recurrence. Another patient described receiving a low

Oncotype DX score but proceeded to chemotherapy because of the size of her tumour. For other patients, results could be flexibly interpreted, particularly patients with scores in a 'grey area'; for example, an intermediate result could justify stopping chemotherapy early due to unpleasant side-effects, as was the case with two forum users.

In these situations, the complexities of Oncotype DX did not always resolve uncertainty but raised questions and worries, sometimes making grey areas larger rather than smaller. These included situations where, long after the test had been conducted, patients continued to wonder about their prospects of recurrence. For example, in an interview with Wendy, conducted three years after her diagnosis, she told us she was not sure what the Oncotype DX test was, and 'never really asked', although she described herself as 'somebody who wanted to know as much as I possibly could'. Having gone through treatment and now being back at work full-time, Wendy explained why she never asked about the test:

> I looked it up online later, I did find out quite a lot although it didn't go into detail about exactly what the test was. And it's quite interesting because I never really asked because I could never work out how to find the right words but I never asked whether, if it came back saying you won't benefit from chemotherapy, is that because the tumour is unlikely to spread or is that because it won't respond? Do you see the difference?

Wendy had received a low risk of recurrence score and had accepted the recommendation to forego chemotherapy, but she remained fearful of recurrence, a common feature of living with or beyond cancer, as poignantly discussed by Horlick-Jones (2011). She remained unsure about whether her low score was due to the fact that 'the tumour is unlikely to spread' or 'because it won't respond' to treatment.

The introduction of the test to already complex diagnostic and treatment pathways created additional distress for some women. Several accounts attributed this to the fact that gene-expression profiling exacerbated the 'rollercoaster' experienced during initial diagnostic processes, with all this 'thrown up in the air' by the introduction of Oncotype DX (breast cancer charity forum), especially due to the time required to wait for the results from the US (up to two weeks). Echoing Gillespie's (2012) findings of 'measured vulnerability', a few participants told us that discussions about the test exacerbated their concerns about their cancer, including Bethany, discussed above, who was diagnosed with breast cancer at the same time as three of her friends. As the only one who was offered Oncotype DX testing, she questioned what this meant about the severity of her cancer as compared with others. Another patient, Chrissy, a woman in her sixties who detected a lump that led to diagnosis, also told us that gene-expression profiling raised a lot of questions for her about why she was being offered this test: 'Who debates whether it, it gets sent off or not? Who ... makes that decision? The consultant or ... I've got a friend that's got tongue cancer ... that's not gone off for any testing. Why ... me? (laughs) Why has mine gone off?' When she was told to have chemotherapy, Chrissy said she was 'shocked' as she expected to go back to normal life after the surgery. Chrissy related her anxieties about the test to the fact that the test was 'something new', and processed in a laboratory in the United States:

> So when they said they were sending samples to America, it was like, well, this is something new, something I don't know anything about ... you'd tend to think if it's a well-known test they would be doing it in this country as well. So it was a bit of ... an alarm bell ringing I suppose as to ... what's different that they need to send it away to do this?

Here the 'newness' of the test was a source of concern rather than a sign of its value. For some this was due to their unfamiliarity with the test and its mechanism. Participants were given a variety of levels of explanation about the technology by their clinician, and engaged with further information about the test in varying ways. The way the test might be used as a cost-cutting mechanism, denying patients treatments they might want, also occasionally came up, as in this quote from Ally, whose plans for an active retirement had been blighted by her cancer:

> So then you start to think, knowing the NHS, knowing the state of budgets, whether that [drug] is not going to be [given], because you do hear in the news don't you, that some people could benefit from having a certain type of drug for any particular condition, but because it's expensive, 'oh we can't give that'; that isn't rolled out to everybody just yet.

Other interviewees did not engage with detailed information around the test, including patients who said they did not possess detailed knowledge of the different tests they had received or the implications of their results. Valerie, a young woman in her thirties, experienced her cancer diagnosis and treatment as 'like a conveyor belt'. She had conducted her own research about breast cancer following her diagnosis, and involved her husband in the processes of treatment decision making following her Oncotype DX result. However, she remained unclear about how the result of the Oncotype DX test was achieved, and what this represented. She explained: 'I've found out various bits and pieces in the booklet that, that it goes to California ... I think it's difficult 'cause ... everyone is clearly different with whether they want to read anything or not. I didn't really want to read anything.'

Here Valerie draws attention to an experience related by many of the patients we interviewed across our wider research, for whom being a responsible patient meant avoiding 'too much' information, limiting their internet searching and the questions they asked, and taking their cancer management 'one step at a time'. In the case of Oncotype DX, this resulted in some women and their loved ones engaging with minimum information about the test, because of the complexity and the amount of information they could take on board at this distressing time. Two patients signalled that they had only engaged with the test because they were required to make a choice, although it would have been, in the words of Alice, 'easier' if her clinician had initially given a clearer recommendation about chemo-therapy, rather than offering her a treatment choice. For these patients, a strong sense of trust in their clinician's assessment of the Oncotype DX result, in the context of other information, rather than the score alone was more significant than the intricacies of the test, highlighting the enduring importance of clinical judgement for patients (Latimer et al. 2006; Bourret et al. 2011).

Conclusion

Oncotype DX was totemic of advances and further personalisation of cancer care in the future across policy, practitioner and patient accounts. While there were a range of views about the clinical utility of the test and its cost-effectiveness, there was nonetheless general support for the role of such technologies in an unspecified future. More pragmatically, the test was commonly associated with greater certainty, and relief for cancer patients from the burden of toxic chemotherapy, or else as providing compelling support for such therapy. Savings and efficiencies in the NHS were highlighted by some as key benefits of the technology being more widely adopted. Practitioners and patients told us the test was valuable as a means of confirming decisions and obtaining reassurance, providing more certainty that enabled them to act responsibly in making wise decisions about the need for treatment to decrease the likelihood of recurrence.

Nevertheless, its promise in practice was muted. There was scepticism, uncertainty and resistance to its wider use, from practitioners choosing not to perform the test as they considered it costly and unnecessary, to patients finding that results did not deliver certainty and reassurance, raising further anxieties and questions (see Ross et al. 2019). At times, patients resisted the impetus to actively research and engage with test results as a means of navigating their illness, and instead sought to limit their engagement with this and other information as a means of maintaining their poise and managing anxiety. The value of the test was thus provisional and in-the-making, as practitioners and patients navigated its implications and experimented with its uptake and interpretation. Being a responsible practitioner or patient could involve a range of orientations towards the test and its results, and choreographing these orientations involved articulation work in the clinic and beyond.

The approvals process was guided by a precautionary logic where uncertainties and scepticism about benefits were given weight, but we found that much of the flexibility and ambivalence we encountered in our study was absent from public discourses about the utility of the test. Although capturing patients' investment in the test and the value it brought to their experiences of treatment, policy and media accounts did not often capture the uncertainties and grey areas that can abound for patients who have been tested, even when certainty is promised or anticipated. Patients' and practitioners' ambivalence was overlaid with more totemic, anticipatory regimes of personalised medical futures, even in processes which purported to question the value of the test and aimed to capture a broad range and variety of experiences to guide policy formulation. The arbitration of contested and conflicting evidence from trials and patient and clinician testimony resulted in continued valuing of the test within the NHS, thus ensuring both that the commercial imperative and the promise of precision medicine continued apace.

Through these dynamics, our case study of Oncotype DX reveals that the promise of personalised medicine is highly contingent and flexible and enacted through articulation work backstage of policy and public discourses. This promise is nevertheless amplified in frontstage policy, advocacy and media framings which assert benefit at the same time as they tend to mask ambivalence. These processes also frame personalised medicine as mainstream, even as the technologies at its forefront may be rejected or become folded into the complexity of responsibilities and decision making involved in the navigation of cancer diagnostics and treatments by practitioners and patients.

Notes

1 www.nature.com/subjects/gene-expression-profiling (accessed 20 June 2020).
2 www.nice.org.UK/guidance/dg34/chapter/1-Recommendations (accessed 20 June 2020).
3 https://breast.predict.nhs.UK/predict_v1.2.html (accessed 20 June 2020).
4 www.nice.org.UK/guidance/dg34/chapter/4-Evidence (accessed 20 June 2020).
5 www.cancer.gov/news-events/press-releases/2018/TAILORx-breast-cancer-chemotherapy (accessed 8 October 2019).
6 www.nice.org.UK/guidance/dg34/chapter/1-Recommendations, section 1.1 (accessed 1 July 2019).

3

Molecular profiling for advanced gynaecological cancer: prolonging foreshortened futures

Commercially produced genomic tests for cancer diagnosis, prediction and treatment are being incorporated into NHS care, albeit unevenly and with much contingency in practice. A range of genomic tests are under research and development as part of the widening diagnostics market: a recent report estimated that the tumour-profiling market would be worth \$12.4 billion by 2024, with genetic biomarkers accounting for the largest share.[1] Companies are producing suites of tests for different cancers and/or tests which work on multiple cancers. For example, Oncotype DX, discussed in detail in the preceding chapter, is now part of a wider set of tests called Oncotype IQ manufactured by the parent company Genomic Health, including tests for other kinds of breast cancer, prostate and colon cancer.[2]

This chapter investigates the development of one such molecular profiling test that has the potential to guide future management of locally advanced or metastatic cancer, but is not yet fully embedded in standard NHS care. Exploring how smaller-scale clinical research creates and prepares the way for further public/private partnerships to deliver personalised medicine, we focus on a feasibility study in an NHS hospital for a commercial molecular profiling test developed by a US company that we are calling Virtue. The multi-platform profiling test can guide treatment decisions for locally advanced or metastatic, gynaecological cancers.[3] First, we look at how the feasibility study was part of building an evidence base for molecular tumour profiling in gynaecological cancers and cancers more widely, and the kinds of value making this involved. This traversed efforts to attain precision and actionability and negotiate the place of commerce with a view to the health service of the future. Secondly, we explore the experiences of patients involved in the study and how they and their family members navigated this experimental space, making sense of the benefits and limitations of the study and associated test as part of their wider cancer experience. We explore the promise of this study, routinely called a trial by the practitioners and patients involved, and the kinds of uncertainties and ambiguity this could bring for patients and their families even as they 'add more evidence into clinical practice' (Metzler 2010). Focusing on patients with advanced or metastatic gynaecological cancer also gives us insights into a different set of experiences from those of ER+/HER2–/LN– early-stage breast cancer patients discussed in the previous chapter. These patients are often older and have experienced cancer for longer, affording different kinds of investments in the future and engagements with new technologies and the certainties they promise. In short, they have a poor prognosis, have already experienced recurrence and are running out of treatment options.

We draw on multiple sources of data to build this case study, including news reports, commercial websites, online patient forum discussions, policy documents, interviews with 16 gynaecological cancer patients who participated in the study, and seven of their family members, conducted in 2017, and three practitioners who ran the feasibility study, interviewed in 2018 and in 2019, when we followed up with them about the results. Before we explore patient and family member accounts, we first look at the ways in which the test can be seen as part of 'a new era for cancer survival' for metastatic and advanced patients (Nawrocki 2018), focusing on the kinds of companies involved in this bioeconomy and the ways they work with clinicians. We go on to consider how Virtue's test, currently only available privately outside of research studies, is being configured for entry into the NHS via this feasibility study (which we are calling VGT), setting out the negotiations around evidence performed in this experimental space.

Precision oncology for advanced gynaecological cancers

A swell of activism has recently grown around gynaecological cancers, historically regarded as a 'Cinderella cancer' (Jasen 2009). Gynaecological cancers, including womb (uterine and endometrial), ovarian, cervical, vulval and vaginal cancer, are more common in post-menopausal women in the UK, with the exception of cervical cancer, which tends to affect younger women more. Although womb cancer is the most common of these cancers, it is ovarian cancer that is the most visible in gynaecological cancer activism, with an increasing number of ovarian cancer charities involved in 'knowledge activism' (Rabeharisoa et al. 2014)[4] as public awareness of symptoms is still relatively poor globally and in the UK in particular. Survival rates have not improved greatly and diagnosis often comes late. We interviewed several ovarian cancer patient advocates during our research. These people were endeavouring to raise the profile of ovarian cancer, to ensure that ovarian cancer patients were not 'left behind' while resources went to more common or more high-profile cancers, such as breast cancer. They also saw themselves as playing a role in educating women about its symptoms and to make sure these were taken seriously.

The challenges faced by ovarian cancer patients were compared to those of other cancers, where improvements had already occurred. As a young patient advocate and statistician, Rebecca, who was diagnosed with a rare type of ovarian cancer in her thirties, commented:

> it really annoys me, like, on Facebook ... your ten friends, 'I'm hosting this for breast cancer' ... I'm thinking 'oh god, why don't you just tell the woman the symptoms rather than, you know, have some of these chain emails that people just do?' ... there's always something for breast, what about ovarian or ... not all the cancers are in, are pink, there's other colours ...

These concerns about a lack of support for and awareness about ovarian cancer meant that Rebecca was particularly invested in social media campaigns such as Everything Teal. She was also optimistic about the prospects of a breakthrough in precision medicine research:

> I reckon in about the next ten years ... hopefully we'll have a break-through or ... perhaps if we could just ... get more funding and get more like what breast has done because breast has had such a significant increase in survival rate ... I know no cancer's nice, but that's more like the gold standard of thing where I've got more the Cinderella type of cancer ...

Many tests offering personalised genetic information are marketed directly to consumers – 23andMe being the best-known of these platforms. Direct-to-consumer genetic testing covers everything from ancestry, traits and characteristics to polygenic risk screening for susceptibility to disease (Hogarth and Saukko 2017). This is part of a process of what Metzler has called 'biomarketization' where biomarkers take increasing salience in the prediction and diagnosis of disease (Metzler 2010; see also Hogarth and Saukko 2017; Prainsack 2017). Companies specialising in molecular tumour diagnostics are particularly focused on developing links with private and public healthcare providers to deliver their tests, given the need for expert analysis of results in a clinical context. This means they must find ways to work alongside or in line with clinical practice and in-house hospital pathology services which have a long history of testing genetic and other biomarkers as part of diagnosis and prognosis, and of meeting stringent research governance processes within public institutions.

There are a number of larger companies in this market, including Illumina (see Chapter 5), but many companies in this sector are smaller and relatively young. Ranging in size and configuration, the companies typically offer a range of services and/or tests framed in terms such as cancer diagnostics, personalised healthcare, functional precision medicine and/or precision oncology. Their websites feature a range of patient and practitioner testimonials in the form of case studies and short films, similar to direct-to-consumer genetic testing services (Arribas-Ayllon et al. 2011). An example of this is Guardant Health's film about Guillermo, a man in his forties from Chicago with metastatic stomach cancer.[5] The film tells us how Guillermo's doctor ordered a range of molecular tests when he came to him for his (third) opinion, at a point where he was very unwell and only had a short time to live. The Guardant 360 proved to be crucial as the cancer showed the EGFR marker (EGFR amplification) and enabled the clinical team to target treatments which dramatically improved Guillermo's health and well-being. Even though this is not a cure, the film offers hope that the team will be able to offer new therapies when his disease progresses and 'get back on top of it'. Tests like these are part of controlling the disease by trying to anticipate drug responses in order to find further, more targeted options to stifle the disease's progression, hopefully extending life and quality of life.

UK patients do not access molecular tests in the same way as US patients such as Guillermo, as most treatments are provided as part of NHS care. In England many of these tests are performed by a network of regional laboratories as part of the Genomic Medicine Service, which specifies which genomic tests are commissioned by the NHS in England, the technology by which they are available, and the patients who will be eligible to access the tests in a National Genomics Test Directory.[6] A national whole genome sequencing service has also been developed in partnership with Genomics England, following on from the 100,000 Genomes Project discussed later in Chapter 5. At the time of writing there are only two commercial tests listed in the directory – Oncotype DX (Chapter 2) and Prosigna, another test that detects the risk of certain types of breast cancer recurring.

UK patients paying for private healthcare can obtain tests not available as part of NHS care, or access them via private health insurance; others can only access tests via research studies (Moore et al. 2019). Diagnostic companies have therefore formed a range of partnership arrangements with private healthcare providers in the UK to facilitate uptake of the tests and to build the evidence of benefit required for licensed practice. For example, Cambridge-based Oncologica® UK Ltd (established in 2014) recently announced a partnership with 'a leading UK private medical insurer' that allows funding of the Oncofocus® cancer test. The company's press release notes that customers who meet agreed clinical criteria will be able to access the test, which will inform the selection of targeted therapies.[7] This includes patients with advanced common cancers not responding to standard treatment, cancers for which there is no standard therapy and carcinoma of unknown origin. Analysing the DNA and RNA extracted from routine biopsy samples, Oncofocus® profiles 505 actionable mutations linked to 700 targeted therapies and immunotherapies that are approved or under trial.[8]

Research partnerships with NHS clinicians are also crucial to this developing market, not just because there are many more patients being treated in these settings than in private healthcare in the UK, but because partnerships of this sort build connections with clinicians who can be important advocates for the test in evaluation and appraisal processes for its wider uptake in the NHS, based on their expertise and experience in using it in practice. This is especially important in the case of molecular diagnostics, as although improved overall survival with lower weekly healthcare costs resulting from molecular profiling for advanced/metastatic cancer patients have been reported in the US (Haslem et al. 2018), the evidence base for benefit is limited in health systems such as that of the UK (Nawrocki 2018). The longer-term benefits of targeted treatments are also difficult to establish in this group, as many patients relapse after a couple of years on the drugs (Marquart et al. 2018).

Virtue's VGT: case study

Virtue is a US-based company with a European branch and international 'partners' in countries such as Australia. It provides multi-platform molecular profiling for several cancer types. The test, which we are calling VGT, has been developed to identify molecular biomarkers that can help to target treatments for metastatic cancer, using a range of tumour-profiling techniques to analyse protein, RNA and DNA in a sample of the tumour tissue.

As the clinical oncologist who coordinated the VGT test told us in an interview, Virtue is 'a company relatively small in the grand scheme of pharma but it's one of many start-ups that have offered similar things'. Virtue's online promotional materials include patient testimonials and links to films, information about the expertise and technologies involved in its platform, and the steps involved in developing personalised recommendations for each patient. Emphasis is placed on the breadth and power of molecular evidence and analysis to give precise results. Patient testimonials include a film featuring an older woman who has been living with cancer for over a decade, thanks in part to molecular profiling provided by Virtue which helped tailor her treatments. The patient praises the company for its support through the process and emphasises how thankful she is for the extra time that the tests have given her. She speaks of her sense of duty to advocate for other patients and how rewarding this has been. This film is part of a set of other patient films, all of which involve patients with metastatic or recurrent cancer who have benefited from this test after standard care options had been exhausted. The section with information for patients on the company website invites patients and family members to share their stories too, alongside details of physicians who have previously ordered the test and guidance on payment arrangements.

VGT is currently only available privately in the UK and is not yet approved as part of standard care in the NHS, although it is accessible to some patients enrolled in research studies and trials taking place in NHS hospitals. Some private health insurance companies also cover VGT on a case-by-case basis. NICE has synthesised the limited evidence of benefit in a briefing document to support NHS commissioners and staff, including contributions from specialist clinical commentators with experience of using the test and of the study we researched. As is common with many such tests, some evidence suggests that the test does contribute towards improved outcomes for patients, but there are no randomised controlled trials or studies of particular cancers to confirm this and no evidence of cost-effectiveness. Most of the studies cited were prospective and non-randomised, comparing VGT-guided therapy with what clinicians said they would probably have done if it had not been available.

We first learned about the feasibility study of Virtue's VGT test when we interviewed the principal investigator (PI) for the study, at the end of a wide-ranging interview in which he discussed his clinical experience with patients and his wider university and NHS roles. The study was part of a number of activities in which the PI was involved, focused on digital technologies in healthcare or what he called 'next generation informatics' in the NHS, evoking the power of 'big' data linkage across the region and institutions via the innovation of large, complex healthcare platforms incorporating a range of biological and social data.

The PI mentioned Virtue after we spoke about our plans for further interviews with patients and offered to help us organise access in the hope that we would be able to conduct 'exit interviews' with patients on the VGT study and feed our results into the overall evaluation of the test. Here we became recruited into the mission of improving personalised medicine for patients, albeit in a loose and unstructured way. We were also told that the VGT study came about through serendipity, when the PI met a Virtue representative at an international meeting and a discussion about how to generate evidence of the 'cancer outcomes' following the test ensued. The PI and Virtue subsequently went on to work together to design a single-centre study and source funding for the work. Initially, they planned to do a prospective study for cancers of unknown primary origin, but this presented logistical problems and would have required them to work at scale, with a budget beyond the scope of funding available. The company was also unable to provide its test for free during the study, given that it was a small company without significant resources. As the PI explained: 'that meant that we did the study as part of routine care and it was very much can the clinicians in the clinic just enter the data and do the testing and see how it influences the management decisions that were taken'; but it still 'felt like we were at the real cutting edge of molecular testing'. As a result, the study was designed to assess the feasibility of NHS adoption of VGT in the treatment of women with gynaecological cancers.[9] Virtue's solid tumour biomarker testing uses a range of tumour-profiling techniques to analyse protein, RNA and DNA in the tumour. A formalin-fixed paraffin-embedded biopsy was sent to Virtue's laboratory in the USA for analysis. Virtue's proprietary algorithm generates a patient report recommending a course of action, which is sent electronically to the clinician within 14 days to inform clinical decision making. NHS England funded this evaluation through a Regional Innovation Fund, which aims to 'support and promote the adoption of innovation and the spread of best practice across the NHS'.

According to the protocol, the study was categorised as a safety/efficacy study with modest purpose, as the clinician who coordinated this study explained: 'It was a pilot study to look at whether this is feasible within an NHS environment ... whether it could theoretically lead to any benefits to the NHS in terms of costs and to see what the costs where of offering a commercial molecular profile.' 'Ironing out' adequate logistics included collaborating with the pathology department and handling specimens from packaging, labelling and sending off, to record keeping. Crucially,

> a patient would firstly need to be relatively asymptomatic ... we would have to send their tumour off to America ... it would be profiled and we'd get the tumour sample back with a molecular profile. So, to do that, the patient needed to be able to wait twenty-eight days to get their next lot of chemotherapy.

The team were interested in what this would mean for patients, if it would be detrimental and if it was acceptable.

In trying to test and improve logistics the team were researching and innovating technical, bureaucratic and cultural as well as molecular processes of personalisation. Clinical participation also had to be facilitated through the study design, as the coordinator explained:

> one of the difficulties in, is that the … profile still requires a certain amount of interpretation because you, you get an answer in the sense that you get a green box that says 'Recommend this drug', or a red box that says 'Don't recommend this', and a grey one that's neutral. But actually, you have to be fairly confident … in trusting that profile and the evidence on which it's based. And, of course, I guess one of the things that's difficult is … empowering the clinicians to be confident about that.
>
> So if you've got a consultant who knows the area well, as all of the consultants will, then they will know that they're recommending three drugs based on trial A, B and C, and they'll be able to tell you about A, B and C. They'll be able to sit a patient down and tell them about A, B and C and how many patients responded and for how long, on average. With this profile, they get a green box, a, a grey box and a red box and a list of preferences, some of which apply to that cancer and some of which apply to other cancers. And so their ability to have an oversight of all of that, I think, is very low. And so that's … a different way of working for the consultants and meant that there was a lot of discussion between them about what was the right thing to do.
>
> Now, actually, we took a lot of the risk from that away in terms of they weren't prescribing drugs that they wouldn't be prescribing anyway … All of the drugs were already available to that patient. I'd imagine it'd be a lot more difficult if that wasn't the case [pause], if that makes sense.
>
> So it's an entirely different level of evidence to a gold standard randomised controlled trial … which makes it very difficult. And so that's where I talk about sort of there was lesser risk in ours because we're only using things that have come out of a gold standard randomised controlled trial.

Trusting the 'black box' of the algorithm for clinicians reliant on seeing and interpreting evidence from clinical trials was thought likely to be difficult, so the study team limited the treatments the profile recommended to drugs and associated trials that the clinicians were already familiar with in order to inculcate trust in the study and to derive value from it. Making evidence-based medicine more explicit, ensuring clinician buy-in and reducing risk by prescribing drugs that have already gone through an approvals process to establish evidence of benefit allowed the study to focus on how to work in and with a limited range of grey areas.

The feasibility study generated uncertainty and interpretation work for clinicians. But coordination also involved negotiating uncertainties about the quality of evidence going into and being produced by the feasibility study itself. For the coordinator, who worked with the PI, this involved managing their own lack of understanding of the link between algorithm and evidence, as in the extract below:

> **Could you, could you explain the ... nature of that literature being cross-checked?**
>
> I can and I can't ... So (laughs) ... from my understanding of the algorithm, it would, if you like, just go through PubMed and say, well, let's say someone's got over-expression of HER2, which is a particular marker on the cells that's commonly known from breast cancer ... and it would then look through the literature and look for manuscripts that ... abstracts ... it would look at drugs that are most likely to cause a response or toxicity or any relevant outcome in cells with HER2 expression, or tumours with too much HER2. It would do that, from my understanding, in patient series trials but also in [laboratory studies] as well.

It also involved accepting limits in the quality of evidence being collected. As the coordinator also noted, the study team could not do a full study of cost-effectiveness, but could instead 'provide a signal for benefit' by collecting a range of data on health economics, outcomes (progression-free survival), quality of life, toxicity and technical data (time to send and retrieve sample), which has not been published at the time of writing. He continued: 'it's difficult to empower patients with this, I think, because we haven't yet reached a level where we have the evidence base to empower the clinicans'. The study was nevertheless considered to be valuable because generating signals of benefit was a small contribution towards the development of a better evidence base, creating the conditions for better-powered research in the future.

As well as managing uncertainties among clinical colleagues about the value of the test and the study to generate incremental and modest value for the field of personalised medicine, the coordinator also had to manage patient expectations where the perceived value of the study could be much higher. The coordinator told us they had to field requests to participate from patients being treated elsewhere. These patients had learned about the research from sites such as clinicaltrials. gov or the CRUK website and included some patients who were planning to pay for the test privately and were willing to travel to be part of the study. The study only had ethical approval to include 'local patients', so these requests were declined. The coordinator drew on these experiences to express concern that the proliferation of studies and trials which only some patients could access, either because they were fortunate to be treated in centres where more trials were running or because they were wealthy enough to be able to travel, would lead to inequities for patients. This was linked to a set of worries about the complexities of cancer and over-promises to patients, 'matching' the 'promise and hope with this new approach to cancer … that patients hear a lot about in the media' with 'the reality of medicine'. In a similar vein to the oncologists interviewed for Chapter 2, the coordinator expressed scepticism about 'hype': 'part of me wonders … whether the proliferation in things like molecular profiles and so on [have] … moved so far ahead of where the evidence is to catch up that, that has its own risks':

> we don't understand key bits of the study of biology to shape it yet … for [Virtue] we may, for instance, have sent off an ovarian tumour sample from straight after their chemotherapy … but that tumour sample may have different markers to one two months later. We don't yet understand how that changes … there's so much complexity now…

In these reflective excerpts the coordinator manages uncertainties to get buy-in for the study while at the same time dealing with excessive expectations and what they framed as patients' need for certainty.

This gives us an insight into the ongoing work of negotiating expectations of personalised medicine for clinicians involved in these kinds of local small-scale studies or trials, including reflecting back on the worth of studies in which they have played a part. The nurse involved in recruitment to the study also looked back on how patients responded to requests for participation, emphasising their positivity and hope, and praising the staff involved:

> I think we maybe had one patient who declined it. They were all quite excited by it. They all thought, you know, this is going to benefit

me. I need – I want to be involved with this. ... so it was ... usually a positive ... discussion with the patient ... and they were very interested. Some of the patients asked to take a copy of their report away ... presumably they – they couldn't understand it fully but – but they want – you know, they were very interested in it.

What made them ... expect to ... benefit ... from [the profile]?

I think the gynae consultants are very good at ... explaining ... I've sat in with quite a lot of consultants over the years, and registrars as well. And some are better than others. But I think the gynae team are very good at explaining. And I think probably from – that they understood what ... they were being told and what they were being asked to do. And that ... potentially by identifying biomarkers ... in their blood we could see which treatments would ... help and which ones probably wouldn't help ... there's a range of treatments you can have for ovarian cancer. And some of them, the ... response to treatment rate is quite low; you know, less than 25%. ... they felt that they'd have more control perhaps over their [pause] over their treatment and decision making, And their ... clinician would have more information how best to treat them, of course.

In this account the nurse underlined the value of participation in the study for patients as a key outcome, focusing on their willingness to participate and apparent sense of control as valuable in their own right and linking this to the skills of the clinicians involved in the study. The lack of opportunity to otherwise access more targeted treatments was also mobilised as a key reason why this test was experienced as valuable by patients.

In the next section, we focus more closely on how patients accounted for their participation and experiences of VGT and the benefits it brought. As we shall discuss, this included accounts of optimism, control and enthusiasm for the test offering more specific information and opportunities for tailored treatments. These positive accounts and expectations were, however, tempered by experiences of unmet expectations in some cases. For other patients, their accounts of expectations and/or experiences of the test and the study were much less positive. To make sense of these themes and this diversity, we explore how genomic approaches such as the VGT study were incorporated into patients' different approaches to uncertainties provoked and at times resolved by the test as part of crafting foreshortened futures. We explore how these tests offered some kinds of certainties but also generated uncertainty and ambivalence; we also consider when the test did not have resonance or meaning for patients, particularly patients who were not invested in future-crafting beyond the day-to-day. However, we also show how engaging with the test enabled these advanced cancer patients to hope for 'other things' even when their personalised results did not significantly impact on their treatment and prospects. This included being part of a bigger future via their research participation.

Patient accounts of participation in the VGT study

Practitioners in our study were keen to underline the benefits of the test and the study for patients facing foreshortened futures and limited treatment options. But in other respects, as in the discussions with the coordinator above, they were concerned about unrealistic expectations among patients because of a lack of evidence of benefit. Clinicians and patients were routinely operating in conditions of uncertainty in the clinic, and in this particular study, but the test offered hope of finding treatments to which the patient would respond well. It was, however, far from universally valued, and patients were elsewhere being cautioned by professionals and patient advocates about uptake of these tests because of a lack of evidence of benefit, albeit within an overarching regime of anticipation of benefit in the future. For example, in a cancer charity forum thread discussing two different commercial tumour-profiling tests, including Virtue's, one of the moderators noted a lack of randomised control trial evidence of benefit, or evidence of benefit in particular cancers rather than cancer in general. Although welcoming the tests as a positive development, the moderator noted their cost and difficulties with interpreting the results to guide treatment decisions.

As we mentioned earlier in the chapter, we were enrolled into this accretion of evidence when we were invited to interview patients who participated in the VGT study by the PI. We were also steered away from observing consultations with patients where the results were discussed, given the potential sensitivities of these consultations and the logistics of being in the right place at the right time. The research nurse who was in charge of the VGT study informed us of the dates of outpatient appointments for patients who were participating in the feasibility study (72 patients in total); we waited to be introduced to the patients by the oncologists, typically after the consultation. Oncologists only mentioned our study to their patients when they felt it was appropriate to do so. We approached 21 patients and, as noted above, interviewed 16. Five patients either declined to participate or were unable to be interviewed due to ill health. Ten interviews were conducted on NHS premises, arranged to coincide with their hospital visit if possible, and six interviews were conducted in patients' homes because it was more convenient for them. During these interviews we carried out an in-depth exploration of participants' experiences of cancer and care in general and the feasibility study in particular, including at which point in their treatment they were approached by research nurses, what they expected from the test and their actual experience of it, how the molecular results were discussed, and how treatment decisions were eventually made. We explored what participation in this study meant to interviewees, and how they managed and made sense of the research and clinical encounters in relation to their previous experiences of care and participating in research, and their hopes for the future.

This particular cohort of late-stage cancer patients were 'living *in* prognosis' (Jain 2007) at the time of our study. Many of them had experienced difficult cancer journeys and were in the later stages of incurable cancer or faced a high risk of metastatic recurrence (Roberts and Clarke 2009; Brown and de Graaf 2013). This makes their experiences particularly valuable for investigating aspirations for personalised care and treatments, bringing fresh insights to a literature that is dominated by the experiences of younger, often more active patients or patients with well-researched cancers with a better prognosis, such as breast cancer (see Miller et al. 2014). For the VGT study participants, the priority was keeping cancer at bay with the hope that, in the future, their cancer might become a managed, chronic illness, rather than seeking a cure. Preparing themselves for future treatments was important for patients who had seen their cancer recur. Most of these patients had experienced long-term treatment or multiple cycles of chemotherapy alongside other treatments, so it was also important to secure decent intervals between treatments to recover from treatment side-effects and more importantly to prepare for the next cycle of treatment.

Although a test such as VGT was, for us, an ideal example of implementing molecular personalisation in a research setting, it turned out that it was by no means central to patients' long and complex cancer journeys. Some patients even struggled to recall the test as it faded into a blur of clinical/research encounters. Against this background, we were struck by how participants still managed to generate diverse accounts of the Virtue test. Our research participants expressed different degrees of interest, understanding and knowledge about the science and technique behind molecular personalisation. But instead of focusing on 'mis/understandings' (Dixon-Woods et al. 2007), we try to situate these accounts within their wider accounts of cancer and care.

As cancer becomes more treatable, if not curable, many people are living with advanced or metastatic cancer. In England it has been estimated that there are thousands of people who have survived for several years with the most advanced stage of cancer, according to recent research from Macmillan Cancer Support and Public Health England's National Cancer Registration and Analysis Service (2017).[10] Patients with late-stage cancers have often experienced long and difficult cancer journeys, including delays in diagnosis and other complications such as multiple co-morbidities. Feeling like a 'time-bomb' (Davies and Sque 2002), some of these patients are living with 'contracted time' (Lewis et al. 2016). For many, recurrence is a matter of 'not if but when', as one interviewee in our study put it. For some patients this awareness involves thinking ahead and preparing for the 'multiple future-times' (Brown and de Graaf 2013), trying to be 'one step ahead' of their cancer. But for others extended futures are set aside for living in the near future. For many of these patients, their priority was to make incurable cancer treatable and manageable for as long as possible, protecting and improving their quality of life. In so doing they are navigating a different kind of future than early-stage patients who might hope for cure or lengthy remission.

In what follows, we focus on three major themes that occur across our set of interviews: first, a wide range of promises and expectations as described by patients and family members; secondly, the multiple reasons for disappointment and frustration they had to deal with;

and finally, how for some patients, the VGT study was not as salient as it was for other more active, relatively younger patients.

Promises of Virtue

Virtue held considerable value for many of these patients and their family members with whom we spoke. Dennis described his understanding of the VGT offered to his wife Helen, both in their seventies, as a 'magic formula they were using in America'. Together with his wife, he hoped that 're-testing the biopsy' would suggest a 'better treatment or more appropriate treatment'.

Such hopes were particularly marked among younger patients in our study, for whom Virtue was part of a more concerted effort to access tailored treatments and engage with the possibilities of personalised cancer medicine. These patients told us they were actively searching for trials of tailored treatments and seeking second opinions at teaching hospitals running trials. Researching alternatives to current or proposed treatment was an important strategy for maintaining a future, which included seeking private cancer care or overseas treatment. These patients were not, however, naïve about the promise of cutting-edge tests and treatments, carefully weighing benefits to quality of life against cost or side-effects (for themselves and for their family). This was a relatively solo set of pursuits for some of these patients. Although they supported their fellow patients by making the occasional donations to fundraising efforts, they did not all participate in collective action or support online. One patient, Donna, who was in her fifties, was an exception. A particularly proactive and well-informed patient, Donna was involved with a national ovarian cancer charity and other patient forums, where she told us the VGT study (which she called a trial) came up in discussion:

> I'm also on ... a Facebook site which is just for ovarian cancer ... sufferers and we share information and links to different sites ... it's a comforting site; people really talk to each other ... and they ... might say, 'Oh, ... I'm going on the VGT trial. Has anybody heard of it?' And then we'll all add our comments and – if we've had it and that kind of thing, so that's quite useful ... So when I do the research or when I'm talking to people, people will talk about the VGT trial but they may have been on a different chemotherapy to me ... So I

think there were one or two people but we tend to talk more about the side effects of the chemo rather than the trial itself. So there was something about some of your samples are sent away but then because of what that forum is about it was more about how you feel rather than the trial itself.

This excerpt gives us an insight into hopes about being on a trial, but focuses more on the comfort offered by comparing experiences even when these were different, with the emphasis on managing side-effects and emotions evoked by participation. Donna also told us that doing research, weighing information and archiving information of clinical trials was a source of reassurance:

I do a lot of research and I save quite a lot of links to different trials and I just think well, okay, well, if I start to feel ill again and it comes back I'll click on this one. So I've got a list of different things I can read.

For Donna, and others, participating in research like the VGT study was one small part of a menu of research opportunities for securing her own future, with the added benefit of helping future patients; as Donna said, 'Hopefully it helps me and it should help others as well. So I will try anything really.'

VGT was also experienced by other patients and their relatives as valuable because it offered bespoke care as well as hope. June and her husband Bob told us about their particularly difficult experience with June's previous care team who said there was no treatment they could offer her. For this couple, VGT study participation offered hope where it had previously been dashed. It also meant an extension of personalising care she had already been receiving from her current care team. Bob associated June's participation in the VGT study with the insurance of personalised care:

I say, the only thing that I gleaned from that [meeting with clinician] was that they were going to take more interest in June's case other than put her into the normal – what we used to call cattle market … where the whole process was like a cattle market.

For Bob, the VGT study was a gateway to more experimental and special options as opposed to standard 'written in stone' treatments, and this was a risk they were prepared to take even though he was aware that this meant June would be a 'guinea pig'.

> just going for a regular treatment that they were offering ... there were nothing outside that they could offer you. But my understanding with this is there's a possibility that would be something that would benefit to treat June's condition but it's not necessarily what's already available, it might be a, a trial that you would volunteer to do ... I thought, well, if the outcome isn't so rosy [on] the path we're treading now, and there was any possibility that there was something that could improve the situation, either not guaranteed but possibly it'd be worth taking a chance, you know what I mean, for whatever reason. Whether or not it would be to prove a point that it wasn't going to be successful if ... they did that treatment, but June would [have] been like a guinea pig say, in order to trial this treatment.

This promise of molecular personalisation was also associated with being privileged to be part of a study where only a small number of people's samples were 'sent off to America', in the words of Mary, a patient in her sixties. Mary's cancer was picked up by a routine smear test when she was 57. When we asked her about motivation for taking part in this study, Mary explained:

> They were doing this trial of sending off to America, the tumours that ... I had and they were going to look at it in a molecular genetic level with a view to being able to personalise my treatment ... Of course, if somebody says [that] to you, you're not going to say no are you? And I was told that ... there was only ... about seventy or eighty people in the country that had been ... allowed to have this done.

For other patients, VGT was an improvement on 'standard' forms of cancer care that they experienced. For instance, another associated Virtue with 'individuality' which is opposed to current 'conveyor belt'-like care. Sally, who was diagnosed in her forties and had since experienced multiple recurrences, said,

> treating everybody individual[ly] is a good idea ... it's difficult for doctors, nurses seeing so many people every day, and I suppose it can tend to be, like a conveyor belt, people coming in and you're saying the same thing. Maybe a bit of individuality might be quite a good thing.

Throughout these accounts of promise, the comfort and reassurance of what was perceived to be more personalised care emerge as important values of the test and the study, for patients and their relatives. Futures were being crafted through the experience of care being more advanced and tailored to the individual in the present. For other patients, and in other respects, the experiences of the study were less positive, and involved recognising and managing disappointment, as we now go on to discuss.

Managing disappointment

Across patients' and family members' accounts, it was common that the VGT study was described as not being particularly burdensome. Their participation was framed as requiring minimum effort, such as no extra visits to the hospital as might be the case with other clinical trials, and it was regarded as non-invasive. Participation did, however, bring additional emotional work in other respects, as participants and their families made sense of risks, disappointment with their results, and conflicting expectations and experiences of the study.

Before deciding to enrol on the study, patients had to weigh up the benefits and risks of participation; patients needed to decide, with consultants' guidance, if they were okay about waiting for the results to come back (as it meant a delay in treatment for 4–6 weeks), as the quote from Marjory below illustrates:

> Because you have to delay your treatment so to go on the trial you have to accept that your treatment is going to be delayed by two months – six weeks [to] two months – something like that. So obviously there is a risk but I talked to Doctor [name of oncologist] about the risk and he didn't think that it was a fast growing – so I decided that, and even if it was I still thought, I've got more scientific basis of it working out by going through the trial than I have if we just guess or take an educated guess.

Marjory told us about her scientific background as evidence of her competency in engaging with the scientific aspects of this and other research on ovarian cancer, as she described why she was prepared to wait for the VGT results. However, not all patients were happy about waiting. Another patient, Kate, told us quite a different story. For Kate, waiting for one month was 'a bit tough because I wasn't having any treatment at all and I was aware of the fact that my tumour marker was going up and my cancer was getting worse'. Kate described her disappointment when the results came back,

> I think that's why I was disappointed that it was just the bog standard treatment [that was recommended]. I felt like saying, 'I could've had this a month ago', you know, cracked on and it would've, you know, perhaps caught it a bit earlier I know it's only a month...

Here the value of the test declines when experiences do not match expectations of tailored treatments and the gamble of waiting does not pay off.

Participants also had to find ways of managing disappointments which arose when their sample was not of sufficient quality to generate meaningful results. As with other research we followed, there was a risk of sample failure with the VGT study. For instance, another patient, Sally was told that her sample 'wasn't brilliant'. When we asked how she felt about this she said,

> Well I was a bit gutted really, 'cause I was expecting this miracle thing that was going to happen to me and, you know, but they did get quite a lot of information from it they said, so yeah.

> **Right, could you ... elaborate, what do you mean by miracle? In what sense?**

> ... because it's a personal diagnostic test, I just thought, maybe they were going to find something that they'd not seen before, or something that maybe would work that I've not tried. Maybe I didn't really understand it all properly, but, I don't know, you just, it's just hope I think, just hope, there's always hope.

Sally described how she got some consolation from the fact that they did find 'some good things' which might help future patients.

Participants also told us of their disappointment at options for treatment being discounted by VGT because the patient did not have the 'right mutations'. This could be experienced as part of a series of routes closing off. For instance, we spoke to Donna's husband Ewan when he accompanied Donna for her last radiotherapy session. For Ewan, participating in research meant reversing Donna's bleak prognosis,

> I just know that trials give me a lot of hope because if we're just going along the path of the chemo and the gap is getting less between

the chemo, then you're on the downward slope really. By being on
a trial, who's to know that, you can make that shoot up, that slope.

Despite Ewan's hope, Donna's test results were disappointing, as
Ewan explained:

[W]hen we sent the biopsy away it came back … they're saying, 'Well,
that's not a route that you can take because you don't have the right
mutation.' So you just sort of ignore it then because you're not going
to pursue that route … Like I say … she didn't have the BRCA; she
didn't have the mutation for [VGT] and … she can't have immunotherapy so I don't know whether that's the stage of it or the … condition
… that she's got…

This extract captures another common strategy of patients and family
members handling disappointment when the VGT results did not
turn out to be a gateway to further treatments, focusing instead on
the next steps and 'moving on' to source value from other research,
tests and treatments. Ewan also talked about his efforts to support
and maintain positivity for Donna as part of this process, although
he acknowledged that it was challenging. Ewan said,

I think [pause] for her to deal with it positively, she has to in her
mind I think, still think that it's going to be cured. I don't necessarily
think that, which is difficult in a relationship. So obviously I don't
voice that … at all if I'm honest. I may discuss it with myself.

Ewan's story captures the challenges for many carers as well as
patients, navigating family members' hopes alongside their own,
calibrating how positive and sceptical they can be against each
other's feelings so as not to cause further upset and to maintain
some equanimity.

The appeal of 'precision' promised by the Virtue test also sat at
odds with patients' desires to have a variety of options, as Jean, a
teacher whose cancer had returned and spread to her lung, described:

So it [the test results] did say that paclitaxel was probably not a good
one for me, and that was the chemotherapy that I'd absolutely hated.
That was the one that made me feel really poorly, so … at that point
I was really glad to see that it said paclitaxel wasn't good, because
I thought that meant I'd never have paclitaxel again, but actually
I've realised that's a silly thing to have been grateful for because it

might be one of my only options at some point, so … you want your options as wide as you can really, though I would prefer not to need it again.

Balancing expectations, individually and collectively, to craft value from participation in this or future research involved managing disappointment in the present and retrospectively, as emotions were reviewed and revised in the face of diminishing options.

Other patients described their disappointment about the lack of novelty from the VGT test result, that is, when the test just confirmed that the same treatment as before was the best option, as in the extract below from Tracy, a civil servant who had just turned fifty when we interviewed her:

> I think when, when I first went onto the … trial and then waited for the results coming back, I imagined that'd be this whole big thing of information, that there'd be lots of information there and things that I could be given that I could look through and, and read up. I was a bit disappointed, to be honest with you (laughs), at the end of it when they just confirmed that they were going to give me … the same treatment, I think, that I'd had for the … cancer before. So it's like, well 'hello (laughs), where's the rest of, where's, where's, where's this, where's this encyclopaedia that's coming back then with all these results as to what works, what doesn't work and everything?'

We see the clash of expectations around what was the reality of the study, echoing the promissory discourses around trials more generally, and the realities of a smaller-scale study which was already operating with limited treatment options as part of the incremental approach to ironing out logistics and gathering evidence to find a pathway for adoption into NHS care in the future. However, for Belinda, like others in our study, having 'other options and things … when the disease progressing and gets any worse' that 'would help … further along the line' was a way of keeping their futures open and remaining optimistic.

Participating in the VGT study was a means by which these patients preserved the possibility of future treatment even when it did not directly affect their current treatment. Regarding the test results as reserve for future treatment or a springboard for more cutting-edge treatment (for example off-label drugs or combinations of drugs) gave patients and their spouses hope and offset immediate disappointment about not being given 'more cutting-edge' and novel treatments in the present.

The complexities of accessing drugs recommended by VGT on the NHS could nevertheless generate frustration and disappointment when promises of precision were unfulfilled. For instance, Tracy could not get a particular targeted drug, recommended by the test, until her cancer recurred. She compared her situation to gambling on 'Bully's Prize', referencing a popular darts gameshow from the 1980s, where competitors who gambled their winnings on a star prize and lost were invited by the host to 'have a look at what you could have won'. Tracy elaborated her frustration as follows:

> So it seems a bit ridiculous that I'd have to go through waiting for it to come back again and then go through all my treatment before I could be offered that drug. [...] And from a cost point of view, it just doesn't make any sense to me either.
>
> I was told that you could pay for it privately ... but you'd be looking at about £70,000 a year, and that once you start paying for it yourself, you'd have to continue because the NHS would never pick up the cost. Whereas if you go third line and they start you on it, after twelve months, drug companies give it for free.
>
> So yeah, I did get the information about the additional drug, yeah. It's a bit like Bully's Prize, 'come and have a look at what you could've won,' isn't it, really? (laughs)

Tracy criticised the organisation of care in the NHS and its rules of eligibility for treatments, which was not only frustrating for herself but she also felt was not cost-effective in the long term.

This echoes a more general sense expressed by some patients and captured in the excerpt from the ovarian cancer advocate quoted at the start of the chapter, about VGT being able to deliver tangible benefits given the limited options for gynaecological cancer treatments. One patient, Jean, told us she had learned from her own research that VGT was 'related to breast cancer rather than ovarian cancer', but expressed disappointment that there was much less of an evidence base in the case of ovarian cancer. She was told by her oncologist that 'if you'd [got] breast cancer we would say straight away ... a hormone blocker, but we don't have that set in evidence'. This meant that the interpretation of the VGT results was not as 'black and white' as she expected. This made her realise that 'I don't think it's helped me quite as much as I hoped it would do.' Like many other patients, Jean nevertheless expressed her gratitude and hope for future patients as follows: 'I'm still grateful that somebody's trying it. And presumably they'll build up a bank of research from doing that that will help others as well, which has got to be a good thing.' Jean's framing of her participation being of value to future patients was linked to a strong sense of the value of the NHS and a concern that, left unchecked, pharma could be 'bleeding the NHS to death'. Jean told us she had a solution to the problem of the high costs of genomic medicine for the NHS:

> You cap what drug companies can charge. At the moment I do believe the drug companies are bleeding the NHS to death. That's my belief … I understand they're a business. I understand that and that their raison d'être is about making money for their shareholders, but I wish somewhere in their – in their ethics was something that was about helping people as well rather than their reason for existence to be to make profit. I believe that if there was a cap, if the government put a cap on what they were allowed to charge, the amount of profit they were allowed to make, that that would mean there'd be more money for this kind of thing.
>
> When I was on the trial, one of the things that concerned me was I'm on a trial where they're finding information that might be useful. Will they then charge so much for it that people – that it won't actually be useful? … I think the pharmaceutical companies will bring the death of the NHS at some point, which is very sad … for people in the future and I think it's really, really sad because I think the NHS is one of the most magnificent things that's been set up.

Jean was unusual in the sense that she advanced an overtly political analysis of molecularisation and the need to limit profit and protect the NHS so that future patients could benefit. For other participants who had experienced or were contemplating the prospect of disappointing results, the possibility of helping future patients was also important, although this was expressed in much more general terms, as a kind of consolation, for example: 'if it doesn't help me, it will help others but hopefully it will help me too'.

Through these various rhetorical strategies, personal 'future diso-rientation' (Roberts and Clark 2009) was managed through appeals to 'future patients' by 'hoping for other things' (Ehlers and Krupar

2014) such as helping future generations, as in the quote from Tracy below:

> But I do understand that it will help them in the future, you know, when they know that they've tried that and that hasn't worked. Then they've got other options that are, that are there. I just thought it'd be a lot of information that they'd come back with. And I'm told that it is a lot of information but ... they don't obviously give me all that because that's not going to help me.

Similarly, June and her husband Bob described their understanding of how research works by combining results and how they were part of it – many individual research projects will not work, but each 'failure' helps research as a whole, including themselves.

> [Bob] Yeah, the only downside to that is that if it didn't work they'd know that that's a dead end but they've used you [June] to find that. But having said that, it's worked for people coming behind that they know it's – that route's not going to be available
>
> [June] ... while you're trying all these things, all that information is being pulled ... So that it's going to help other people ... As well as you ... Well, [if it doesn't work] I would go onto the column where it didn't work, into a percentage thing.

The value of participation for June became a matter of helping future patients.

Lack of salience

VGT results had to be processed by patients in relation to an array of treatment experiences and decisions, which sometimes resulted in this particular study blurring into other studies and trials they had previously experienced or anticipated as part of their future. We did, however, encounter a small group of patients for whom the VGT study held very little salience. These were among the oldest patients we spoke to and all faced a bleak prognosis: one patient told us she had reluctantly agreed to receive palliative care to address co-morbidities and other complications, another patient was on third-line chemotherapy, and two other patients were anticipating another recurrence of their cancer. While two of these patients told us that they had a lot of support from their husbands, the other two patients had less support from family members. One of these patients had lost her husband to cancer while she was undergoing her own cancer treatment and the other patient's husband had early-onset dementia.

For this group, putting trust in their care team was particularly important, much more so than embracing the idea that VGT would transform their prospects. Their participation in the VGT study was a matter of trust, and continuity of care was key, with the test slotting into rather than determining these arrangements. These patients were also not as well connected, digitally or otherwise, with other patients due to their limited mobility and/or their stoic inclination to 'desire a private disease experience' (Kaiser 2008: 79). This did not mean that these patients were completely disengaged from gleaning information and doing research. They spoke of the need to 'keep fighting' cancer, and they were doing what they could manage to support that effort, such as regularly collecting newspaper cuttings about new cancer treatments which they might be able to mention to their oncologist. However, the VGT test did not figure in accounts of their current and future care in any detail, and there was minimal engagement with what genomics involved or meant. Instead, a strong emphasis on stoicism or getting through each day was evoked in their accounts, rather than a strongly articulated sense of future, as the following encounter with one of our participants, Maureen, illustrates.

We interviewed Maureen in the chemotherapy unit while she was receiving her infusion. When we first met her at the clinic she was with her husband, but on this occasion she was alone. She apologetically explained that her husband would not have been a great interviewee for us as he has dementia. She added that both her and her husband found the waiting and boredom of a long chemotherapy session difficult, and she struggled to 'entertain him for eight hours' let alone encouraging him to engage in a research interview. In the interview, Maureen focused on her ongoing pain in her lower body and how hard it had been for her to address this, with the VGT test getting only a passing mention. Referencing reduced resources in the NHS, Maureen linked her depleting options with ageist media coverage, as she satirically commented: 'Oh, all these old people are taking up all the beds, they're living too long and they're costing us too much.' Having had a discussion about palliative chemotherapy, Maureen shared her worry about being regarded as an undeserving 'bed-blocker'. For patients such as Maureen, VGT was a secondary part of their efforts to secure the kinds of personalised care they valued and hoped to maintain, a care she was concerned was under threat from rationing and discriminatory interpretations of deservingness.

These accounts sat within a wider narrative of cancer and care where the importance of stoicism was highlighted, which at times made these interviews particularly challenging when the perception was that there was no special story to tell. It was not surprising that two out of the four interviews in this group were the shortest among all sixteen interviews. Both patients' dominant account was of getting on with things:

> It happened. I've got to put up with it. it could've been somebody else. I didn't say 'why me?'... I've always been a very quiet type, a person that just takes it. It's me, that's the way it is.

> [I] just take everything in my stride.

VGT in this context was not imbued with particular meanings or emotional work, as patients concentrated their efforts on managing day to day.

Conclusion

In this chapter we have considered how the feasibility of introducing a novel, commercial, molecular profiling test into the NHS was examined in a research study designed to develop an evidence base for wider implementation, as part of efforts to transform the way the NHS offers profiling and to understand how to make this valuable to patients and clinicians. A range of professionals (including social scientists) were being enrolled in these efforts, alongside patient participants. There were numerous uncertainties around the development of the test and its future in the NHS, just as there were uncertainties for patients and practitioners making sense of test results from which evidence of benefit has to be drawn. The predictive potential of the tests was therefore highly contingent, as was the extent to which the results being produced could prolong or maintain a future for patients with advanced cancers. The promise of precision was therefore vague and underspecified.

Chapter 2 explored the uptake of a genomic intervention in cancer care and its place in practice. This revealed that the technology was far from fully embedded and that its promise was much more contingent than some of the press coverage might have suggested. This chapter has presented further evidence of the conditionality and incrementalism in genomic medicine in the cancer clinic. Although there was a clear impetus to enhance precision and actionability in the case of VGT, its value could be fleeting or unrealised because of the complexities of cancer, health and family commitments. For some patients and their families engagement with the study offered a sense that options were being created or sought out by their care team and, even if no new options arose for them personally, they would arise for patients in the future, extending or transposing the promise of prediction and actionability into the future. For another group of patients, however, the test was not invested with particular promise and the personalised kinds of care they sought were more immediate as they focused on managing their cancer symptoms day to day.

This contingency and flexibility in the use of the test, its results and implications for patients was, of course, a product of professional efforts to find new pathways and protocols for embedding the test into practice, 'smoothing out' processes as well as delivering precision to individual patients. It also extended to the way the study was loosely framed as a trial by both practitioners and patients, and the various different ways the algorithm and the evidence base being developed were described to us as we proceeded with our research.

Through these processes we see the value of the test as something always in the making: value was dynamic in the sense that it was negotiated across place and time and interpreted differently by the actors involved. Practitioners, patients and family members appreciated the value of the test in various ways – ranging from its totemic value of precision and personalisation to its value as a source of reassurance or comfort in the face of uncertainty. But in other respects, the value of the test fell away, as its promise was not realised through the study design or processes (e.g. sample failure) for professionals and for patients who had hoped for something more from their participation. Other kinds of value could sometimes be salvaged from these disappointments and setbacks, including the possibility of benefit for future patients, but value nevertheless retained a precarious and contingent quality and value making required considerable emotional and articulation work from patients, family and practitioners.

In the next chapter we turn to consider how these contingencies and complexities played out in another kind of personalised cancer medicine, focusing on a much larger-scale UK-wide trial with similar aims of developing infrastructure, tackling stubborn cancers, building evidence to make more treatments available for the future, and supporting drug development more widely.

Notes

1 www.prnewswire.co.UK/news-releases/cancer-tumor-profiling-market-worth-12-4-billion-by-2024-exclusive-report-by-marketsandmarkets-tm–801170582.html (accessed 2 July 2019).
2 www.Oncotypeiq.com/en-GB (accessed 2 July 2019).
3 Because of its small scale and specific location the main practitioners involved in the study we explore in this chapter would be easily identifiable if we were to name the test and parent company. In order to preserve anonymity we will use the pseudonym Virtue for the company and VGT for the study.
4 For instance, Target Ovarian Cancer's Pathfinder which is 'groundbreaking research that provides a detailed picture of the experiences of people living and working with ovarian cancer in the UK. The latest Pathfinder will provide a definitive snapshot of the UK's ovarian cancer landscape in 2016.' www.targetovariancancer.org.UK/our-campaigns/pathfinder (accessed 20 June 2020).
5 https://guardanthealth.com (accessed 22 October 2019).
6 The service set up is slightly different in Scotland, with the Scottish Medicines Consortium advising on new medicines. Four regional genetics centres have integrated laboratory and clinical services. The Molecular Pathology Consortium investigates molecular markers for tumours and the Scottish Genomes Partnership is a key pillar of Scotland's Ecosystem for Precision Medicine. See www.scottishscience.org.UK/sites/default/files/article-attachments/Genomics%20Full%20Report.pdf (accessed 20 June 2020).

7 www.oncologica.com/oncologica-collaborates-with-all-leading-health-insurers-to-advance-personalised-medicine-for-patients-with-cancer (accessed 3 April 2020).

8 www.oncologica.com/oncologica-collaborates-with-all-leading-health-insurers-to-advance-personalised-medicine-for-patients-with-cancer (accessed 3 April 2020).

9 https://clinicaltrials.gov/ct2/show/NCT02668913 (accessed 20 June 2020).

10 www.macmillan.org.UK/about-us/what-we-do/evidence/research-funding/our-partnerships/national-cancer-registration-and-analysis-service.html (accessed 20 June 2020).

4

Optimising personalisation: adaptive trials for intractable cancers

We have explored molecular profiling for some breast cancer patients for whom targeted treatments have a longer history than for most cancers, but where the introduction of commercial tests is relatively recent in UK contexts. We have also considered gynaecological cancer patients accessing another commercial test as part of a feasibility study. For other cancer patients, personalised medicine is experienced via a new generation of larger-scale, multi-sited adaptive clinical trials. It is to this platform that we now turn.

As we discussed in Chapter 1, randomised control trials (RCTs), the 'gold standard' of evidence-based medicine, have been superseded by what Keating and Cambrosio (2011) describe as a 'new style of practice' in medical oncology, based on large trials across multiple sites to develop targeted therapies for subtypes of cancers based on genomic profiling. Multi-arm trials test several different treatments at once. If a particular drug is not proving efficacious the trial arm can be closed and new treatment arms brought in (Medical Research Council 2014; West 2017), depending on response and recruitment rates. Trials adapt as results come in, a different methodological approach to traditional RCTs.

Such trials hold out particular promise for patients for whom prognosis is poor and treatment options are few. Lung cancer is an example of one such intractable cancer with very poor outcomes. Patients with lung cancers are typically diagnosed in the late stages of the disease, making it more difficult to treat. Later diagnosis is partly a feature of the difficulties with identifying cancer symptoms, but also a result of the stigma and shame associated with lung cancer in particular, as it is associated with smoking, which may further delay the seeking of help (Chapple et al. 2004). Lung cancer is also associated with deprivation, where smoking rates are taking longer to decline, exacerbating inequalities (Powell 2019). Lung cancer is also difficult to treat due to the late stage of diagnosis, the challenges of surgery (and biopsy) and other difficulties with the health and social circumstances of patients. Genomic research has identified a range of molecular subtypes of lung cancer (EGFR, ALK) suitable for targeted treatments, and both mutations may be tested for during treatment pathways, but prognosis is still poor. The more successful developments of targeted treatments in breast and blood cancers have yet to be replicated in lung cancer, and current national efforts are underway to promote research and develop new targeted treatments.

Multi-site, multi-arm trials are important to building personalised medicine in health services such as the NHS, developing partnerships across centres, regions and with industry, embedding infrastructures of delivery, and investigating how to maximise participation and acceptability among clinicians and patients. Such trials are part of a programme of transformation of healthcare provision to embed personalisation, alongside other larger projects and initiatives such as the 100,000 Genomes Project, discussed in the next chapter.

In this chapter we investigate one such adaptive, multi-arm, multi-site trial for lung cancer, examining how the optimising logic of the trial was enacted and the kinds of value that emerged in the process (Montgomery 2017a; 2017b). We show the ways in which trial leaders, practitioners, patients and family members gave meaning to the promise of the trial and sought to realise value for patients now and in the future. This was clearly difficult to accomplish in practice, and we capture how patients' and indeed clinicians' disappointments and anxieties manifested and were managed, in part, through efforts to calibrate expectations. This included lowering (personal) expectations (Gardner et al. 2015) and cultivating expectations that other patients would benefit in the future instead. In doing so, we draw on an analysis of professional literature, press and website coverage on the trial, as well as observations and interviews conducted between 2016 and 2018. We interviewed 14 practitioners (12 clinicians – including four nurses, three pathologists and two scientists), observed 21 encounters in clinics (two MDTs, two biopsy procedures for the trial, 17 consent meetings for participation in the pre-screening), interviewed five patients who participated in the trial (and two of their family members) and five patients who participated in pre-screening for the trial. We also gathered data from two online forums and platforms where the trial was discussed by patients and their relatives between 2015 and 2017.

Stratified medicine and an adaptive trial

The National Lung Matrix Trial (Matrix) is a multi-site, multi-arm, adaptive trial of treatments for people with lung cancer, based on the molecular profile of their cancer, linked to a pre-screening Stratified Medicine Programme 2 (SMP2). It is funded by Cancer Research UK (CRUK) and run by the University of Birmingham CRUK Clinical Trials Unit in collaboration with the Experimental Care Research Network, NHS and industry partners (initially Illumina, Pfizer and Astra Zeneca). We became interested in researching this trial following discussions with one of the investigators, who was very engaged with precision oncology and saw the trial as a major exemplar of this new approach. With their assistance we were able to develop a case study of the pre-screening component and the trial at one site, which included interviews and observations with staff and patients. We subsequently expanded our case study to include another hospital, partly because it was difficult to recruit patients to our study (there were small numbers being recruited to the trial and patients were unwell, so approaching them to request interviews and observations was not always appropriate). As we will discuss, the trial turned out to be an exemplar of the difficulties with making personalised genomic medicine for cancer work for current patients in treatment.

SMP2 is an observational, pre-screening study, designed to screen up to 2,000 non-small-cell lung cancer (NSCLC) patients in order to identify genetic changes in their tumours. This determines their eligibility for entry into the Matrix trial, where they will be matched to treatments based on the genomic profile of their cancer, and the benefits of these treatments will then be assessed. SMP2 has an additional aim of 'continu[ing] to pioneer the use of next-generation sequencing (NGS) technology in the NHS to prove large scale genetic testing works within the NHS'.[1] The trial, while offering promise to patients, is also preparing the infrastructures and processes to make personalised genomic medicine feasible. This includes the following developments, described on the CRUK website:

> Our Technology Hubs are centralised, quality assured molecular diagnostic NHS laboratories in Birmingham (West Midlands Regional Genetics Service), Cardiff (All Wales Medical Genetics Service) and London (The Royal Marsden). They use innovative NGS technology to detect a variety of changes in a patient's tumour DNA sequence. The NGS panel, consisting of 28 genes, was developed in close collaboration with Illumina, and can be updated regularly to reflect the needs of the programme.

The study design notes:

> The management of patients with non-small-cell lung cancer (NSCLC) has been transformed in the past 10 years. The identification of EGFR-activating mutations as a predictive biomarker for the use of EGFR tyrosine kinase inhibitors ushered in the era of stratified medicine in NSCLC [1]. Only 4 years elapsed between the description of EML4-ALK fusions [2] and the registration of crizotinib for treatment of ALK fusion-positive disease. Alongside these therapeutic advances have been a change in the regulatory landscape; the provisional registration of crizotinib was based on high signals of activity in non-randomized, single-arm studies [3]. A series of publications culminating in the data from The Cancer Genome Atlas (TCGA) for both adenocarcinoma and squamous cell lung cancer have considerably widened the number of potentially treatable targets, albeit in small molecularly defined patient cohorts [4, 5]. Efficient testing of drug–biomarker combinations is necessary in order to unlock the true potential for stratified medicine for NSCLC. The National Lung Matrix Trial (NLMT), funded by Cancer Research UK in partnership with AstraZeneca/MedImmune and Pfizer, includes many of the potentially actionable molecular aberrations identified in NSCLC. (Middleton et al. 2015: 2464)

SMP2 and Matrix followed on from SMP1, a 'proof of concept' study, which involved molecular pre-screening of cancer patients with melanoma, breast, ovarian, lung, colorectal and prostate cancer at eight hospitals to establish feasibility for the NHS and acceptability to patients. They are run via the Experimental Cancer Medicines Centres Network (ECMCN) formed in 2007, with funding from CRUK, NIHR and UK Departments of Health. The network involves 18 adult and 17 paediatric cancer centres to 'assist in the delivery of early phase cancer studies between research partners to enable faster and more personalised patient benefit'.[2]

Presented by the trial website as 'the largest precision medicine trial in non-small cell lung cancer globally',[3] Matrix involves a rolling programme of recruitment to treatment arms which can close and open as knowledge about the effectiveness of drugs develops through the research. In press releases about the trial, the principal investigator (PI), Dr Gary Middleton, based at the University of Birmingham CRUK Clinical Trials Unit, noted:

> This is one of the largest ever personalised medicine trials in any cancer, one which attempts to match the right treatment to the right patient based on an in-depth understanding of what makes their own cancer cells grow and survive.
>
> For our patients, it's a tremendous opportunity to access a wide-range of therapies tailored specifically to their particular type of lung cancer. For people caring for lung cancer patients in the UK, it's exciting to be able to offer these treatments to patients when they're still at a very early stage of clinical development.
>
> With this Matrix trial, cancer medicine in the UK now becomes a key global player in the search for more effective targeted therapies for people suffering from this devastating disease.

As is common in narratives of this sort, the PI emphasises the excitement and promise of the trial and the opportunities it affords patients by giving them access to experimental treatments. The trial is also contributing to the scaling up of UK capacity in the promissory bioeconomy of genomic medicine.

By mid-2016, after it had been running for around a year, the ECMCN reported that the trial had recruited 50 patients, rising to 100 by November that year, with patients receiving one of '8 Investigational Medicinal Products provided within this trial by either AstraZeneca or Pfizer, within 17 of the 21 distinct cohorts'.[4] At this point the trial also received an extension and continues to recruit at the time of writing. Seven of the treatments being trialled during our research were targeted agents (provided by AstraZeneca or Pfizer) with the eighth arm for patients with non-actionable mutations. As the Birmingham University description of the trial notes:

> A secondary objective of the trial is to provide the opportunity for industrial partners to test novel agents in the cohort of patients who

are not positive for any of the actionable targets in the trial, referred to as the no actionable genetic change arm. In particular, if interim analysis shows significant activity for one of the targeted drugs in a targeted group then it may be relevant to assess the putative biomarker specificity of this drug by including it as a treatment option for the no actionable genetic change arm. Such an assessment could be important to inform the design of future trials for that drug. During the course of the trial, any drugs that are selected for allocation to the no actionable genetic change arm will be included in a pipeline of options that become available sequentially. The first drug to be tested in this arm is durvalumab (Cohort NA1).[5]

This multiplied the experimental value of the trial, facilitating opportunities for drug companies and patients to experiment with novel drugs.

By December 2016, 87 out of 107 patients were receiving targeted treatments, and plans were underway to develop two new cohorts with treatments provided by another pharmaceutical partner for other patients. The trial was designed to expand in this way to increase the numbers of patients involved.[6] The trial was also supported by expert review groups to improve the process of obtaining and analysing samples, including via training of appropriate staff: 'Through working collaboratively across disciplines we are committed to improving existing NHS clinical and laboratory pathways to increase the number of molecularly eligible patients identified and subsequently treated with novel targeted therapies.'[7] The importance of developing better processes and technologies was a major theme in news about the trial featured in the ECMCN webpages that give an account of its progress. Although there was considerable optimism about recruitment continuing to improve, with new recruiting centres and treatment arms being opened up, more patients and more 'meaningful results' were still needed for the trial to be a success. This all involves considerable work and engagement from healthcare staff, as well as patients, as the following extract shows:

> SMP2 has recently completed the fifth comprehensive sample and data audit. The team will shortly be distributing audit reports to enable sites to identify areas for improvement. Performance across the network is steadily improving, and their focus now is to challenge sites to test as many patients as possible through SMP2 and carefully track eligible patients through to NLMT. We need commitment and

support from the entire ECMC network to increase recruitment and maximise translation between SMP2 and NLMT, to ensure that this study continues to deliver.

The SMP2 team has been working closely with Illumina, our genetic technology provider and the three Technology Hubs/genetic testing laboratories, to develop a new and improved version of the 28-gene NGS panel. The new version, launched on 20 March 2017, features increased probe coverage, particularly in poorly performing regions, to reduce the gene fail rate and the addition of gene regions to the panel to allow new drug treatments to be delivered via NLMT. These improvements should mean that a higher proportion of patients receive a more meaningful result from their first sample, increasing the number of patients molecularly eligible for NLMT without the need for a repeat biopsy or repeat sample being tested.[8]

Counting the numbers of patients screened in SMP2 (800 patients screened in 2017 'alone') and recruited to Matrix (197 by the end of 2017) was an important means by which the trial leaders sought to establish markers of success in the earlier years of the project (an approach we will also find in the next chapter in relation to the development of WGS for cancer patients as part of the 100,000 Genomes Project).[9] However, after 2017 there is little information on recruitment in the public domain, with the main project website information for patients noting that the aim is to recruit upwards of 600 patients, around 30 per cohort,[10] with the target 'amended throughout the course of the trial with the addition of more treatment arms and cohorts and removal of arms and cohorts showing insufficient signal of activity'.[11] CRUK reports that by November 2018 the trial had recruited 250 patients. There is also a report of high attrition rates between screening and entry to the trial arm (circa 90 per cent), including on social media where we found a slide from the trial entitled 'The inevitability of attrition'. At the time of writing there are eight trial arms, and the non-actionable arm and two other arms have closed.[12] It is also noted that recruitment is expected to end in 2021.

The trial is a prominent example of precision medicine, with the difficulties around recruitment and treatment benefit acting as a spur for further investment and organisational/professional change, rather than as a sign of failure (Hiley et al. 2016). The trial has been framed as a success for the state, cancer charities, professionals and the market. When the Secretary of State for Health, Matt

Hancock, visited a strategic University/NHS alliance in Birmingham in 2018 he learned about this 'ground-breaking' trial.[13] When a deal was signed with the pharmaceutical company Mirati Therapeutics to include its experimental drug sitravatinib in another arm of the trial, its CEO noted that the programme presented an 'exceptional opportunity for clinical research'.[14] In a 2018 *Telegraph* article entitled 'Personalised Medicine "Transforms" Survival Chances in Incurable Cancer' which focused on results from a US study presented at the American Society for Clinical Oncology (ASCO), a CRUK representative explicitly mentioned Matrix when interviewed about the topic:

> Drugs that target changes in a patient's cancer cells have transformed the way cancer is treated, as this study illustrates.
>
> Cancer Research UK scientists are currently advancing this tailored approach via several studies aimed at personalising treatments, such as our National Lung Matrix Trial which is matching lung cancer patients to targeted drugs that will work for them with the ultimate goal of saving more lives by finding the right treatment for each person. (Bodkin 2018)

Through these processes it is not just the trial that is 'rolling' or evolving in terms of recruitment targets and arrangements, treatment arms and funding arrangements; its values also evolve as it is variously presented as, on the one hand, transformative, groundbreaking and part of a new era, and on the other, as part of a more modest process of incremental change and development of services, professional capability and infrastructures. Overcoming the difficulties and challenges of recruitment and attrition becomes part of the process of transformation as the value of the trial is reasserted rather than undermined. The development of new insights into knowledge, actionability, validation processes and valuation measures were also considered successes of the trial, rather than health gains for patients per se. The trial and the programme were, thus, optimised in practice, through efforts to improve treatments for patients, as we now go on to explore in more detail.

Making the trial work

The Matrix trial was often one of the last treatment options for patients following the completion of standard options (usually chemotherapy and/or radiotherapy). Recruitment into and remaining on the trial was challenging, not just because the patient's molecular profile had to match a trial arm that was open for recruitment, but because the sample also had to be of the right quality and the patient had to be well enough to participate and meet a range of other eligibility criteria. The SMP2 pre-screening study was the first step to being part of the trial. At this stage, patients gave their consent for surplus tissue from routine biopsies to be analysed using next-generation sequencing technology. Entry into the trial also required patients to consent to a further separate biopsy procedure to collect tissue to be analysed using next-generation sequencing at a separate institution to direct entry into one of the trial arms. Ensuring that these samples were of sufficient quality and quantity involved considerable articulation work, or 'artful integrations' including configuration and customisation, 'incorporating technologies into everyday working practices and keeping them working' (Suchman 1996: 407).

Enthusiasm and support for SMP2 and Matrix from one of the main investigators and one of the research nurses on the trial enabled us to develop our initial plans to follow patients and practitioners working on the trial at one site. For these actors, Matrix held considerable promise as a new paradigm of personalisation, but it brought with it the challenge of implementation, as one consultant oncologist noted:

> It's taken many years … to bring it into clinical focus … that genomic medicine is important. And I think the things that have really been the tipping points in doing that have always been … market authorisation of … a drug for an actionable mutation, and subsequent cancer drugs fund or NICE guidance supporting its use in, in practice … once they come into place … there's been a headlong rush to try and institute it that wouldn't have been possible if a lot of backroom work hadn't been done for many months or even years …
>
> … a lot of that work of building teams who are flexible and adaptive at the interface between clinical and laboratory medicine … is necessary to get a good … in-house solution to genomic testing. And that can't be turned … on a sixpence when NICE give their guidance.

We also encountered considerable scepticism and concerns about the trial when we engaged with lung cancer practitioners involved in recruitment. This was linked to a general sense of the difficulties of working with very unwell patients, difficulties with implementation and a vague sense of beleaguerment with the bioeconomy of which the NHS is a part. As another consultant noted:

I think the genomics has changed ... threshold for some patients ... by virtue of our own data on what the chance of these mutants is, it's allowed us to have more ... personalised discussion with the patient about whether or not they go for a biopsy, but ... if they don't want it, then they don't get it.

[But] ... our patient cohort ... is quite deprived, low education achievement, low familiarity with medical advances ... I'm sure in a breast cancer clinic that's different, in the lung cancer clinic no one turns up with a Google search or anything like that, or hardly anyone ... we have occasional middle-class patients, but they're few and far between, so no ... the population as a whole is very ... has a very low level of understanding of [genomics]

My concern is the very cosy relationship between pharma and the other ... groups, and the professional groups as well, and I think pharma will often be ... behind the scenes cheering these people on ... when they are in the newspaper ... these are all tragic stories, of course they are, I mean I see these patients every week and it's very sad that you have young ... patients with young families and it's devastating ... but sometimes when you're deciding how to invest limited funds there will always be losers and ... there needs to be a degree of equity across the list in terms of ... who loses out, because there are the people who lose out when expensive things get funded, you just never see them, they're just never there in the papers.

Working in this context was challenging for clinicians trying to give patients the best possible care, and included managing some difficult dilemmas around supporting patients to pay for targeted treatments privately, despite the general view in the team that private medicine was problematic. As one consultant put it, 'I don't want to deal with money.'

Practitioners were engaged in an intricate balancing act to recruit patients on to the SMP2 pre-screening study and access targeted treatments on the Matrix trial, and ensure they were receiving the best possible care at the right time, protecting patients who were too unwell to participate (e.g. having another biopsy), or keeping the trial 'in reserve' for when the initial round of treatments was no longer working, and not raising hopes unnecessarily. Some were sceptical about the value of the study given its complexity and the difficulties with getting a result which would direct entry into one of the treatment arms. Even those practitioners who were more positive, such as the nurses directly involved in recruiting patients to the pre-screening study and caring for patients on the trial, had to navigate numerous difficulties with recruitment, sampling and obtaining results from tumour tissue and managing patient expectations and disappointments. This involved working with a complex mix of organisational arrangements, materials and emotions, while trying to optimise the care of unwell patients with often rapidly deteriorating health.

Several described feeling 'hopeless' about the trial, with others describing it as a 'soul-destroying' process, because of the high attrition in recruitment from the pre-screening study to the trial. This included a series of 'failed' samples which either did not pass quality control to be suitable for analysis or did not produce evidence of genetic changes that would mean that the patient could be recruited to one of the treatment arms of the trial. This led some practitioners to change how they 'sold' the pre-study to eligible patients who could be well enough to participate in Matrix, including managing and, at times, lowering patients' expectations of results being returned that would direct entry into the trial. Not explicitly mentioning Matrix or treatments available on the trial arms was one strategy that was sometimes adopted, illustrated in extracts from fieldnotes below, where two patients were separately being interviewed about consent for SMP2. The first extract follows on from a discussion about where the tissue will go for analysis and what form it will take (a section from a block, to another hospital) involving one of the clinical trials assistants (CTA) responsible for recruitment:

> The CTA goes on to explain that by testing the tissue they're looking for 28 genes, which might help 'further down the line' but also stresses that the patient 'shouldn't worry about this'. The patient nods and agrees, 'yeah, alright, why not,' and doesn't ask any further questions. CTA: 'you're great' (laughs). The patient thoroughly reads through the consent but doesn't ask any further questions – seems more concerned about the CTA having to take blood 'there won't be any left'! Whilst the CTA labels the vial, she asks whether the patient has ever been a smoker, 'yes (looks at me) but I've cut down now'. He describes how his daughter visits him and complains about him smoking – 'we can smell it'! [Sense of shame here.] The CTA ended the

consultation by thanking the patient 'for helping us' and wished him luck with his treatment.

Here we see the CTA downplaying the possibility of SMP2 coming up with results quickly, lowering expectations (Gardner et al. 2015), taking on the burden of worrying about results on behalf of the patient and keeping the encounter focused around the patient's positive outlook and willingness to help.

The process with the second patient is similar:

> The CTA introduced herself and asked, 'did the consultant give you a leaflet about stratified medicine?' The patient explained that he hadn't but she couldn't be sure as her granddaughter deals with most of the information, 'she takes everything in'. The CTA went on to explain what the study entails 'it's looking at the genetics to look at different types of cancer, we send a sample of your tissue to look at the DNA (little bits and pieces) and send to the Royal Marsden for analysis.' The CTA explained that they're looking for 28 genes, which may mean the patient's eligible for research 'further down the line' (the patient nods and agrees). Again, the CTA stressed that the patient shouldn't worry and that if they're eligible the consultant will 'talk this through with them'. The patient is given the opportunity to ask questions but doesn't and just asks about whether they need to do anything 'nasty' to get the tissue sample. The CTA explained that they didn't and that it would just involve sending old tissue along with a blood sample 'one off sample'. At this the patient threw her hands in the air and said 'get on with it, do what you've got to do' and laughs. Throughout the appointment the patient seemed quite passive 'yes, yeah, nodding' and I was unsure exactly how much information they were retaining. The CTA took the patient's blood and I waited by the ECG machine (no chairs). Ending the appointment, the CTA said that she hoped the patient would get some results back but that 'I won't bother you again'! She also thanked the patient who said again how much of an important role her granddaughter plays when accompanying her to appointments etc, 'she's fantastic, does everything'. The patient also told us … her granddaughter is expecting a baby and had just been to do some shopping. Once the patient had left the room and the CTA was finishing the paperwork she said 'that lady's got a great-grandchild on the way, it's so depressing because she'll probably die.' 'People just drop and die and there's no way of knowing. I really think it's all down to DNA; it's a DNA lottery.' 'Along with melanoma it's my least favourite cancer.'

This extract gives us an insight into some of the frontstage and backstage work (Lewin and Reeves 2011) involved in the pre-screening study and its potential as a gateway to recruitment to the trial. Frontstage the work could involve decentring some of the details and purpose of the trial and focusing on the pre-screening study in clinical appointments. This was a means of putting patients and family members at ease, being positive about their future, trying to reduce the burden of involvement (information to be processed, time spent in the appointment) and offering an opportunity for care and expressions of gratitude. Backstage, in team meetings and corridor talk, there were other kinds of emotions – frustration, sadness and disappointment to be managed, given the poor prospects of many of these patients. Staff also had to carefully negotiate approaching patients about the study, resolving conflicts among themselves in the process. For example, we were told patients with brain metastasis (mets) could be entered into SMP2 but they were not eligible for Matrix. This could result in tense conversations between the senior CTA and the consultants. Consultants were reluctant to approach patients with brain mets for recruitment into SMP2 because of how unwell they were and because they would not be eligible for Matrix. SMP2/Matrix were conflated as one study here (SMP2 leading to Matrix), but at times, when eligibility criteria conflicted, the senior CTA had to do a lot of work to convince consultants of the value of recruiting patients to SMP2 despite not being able to enter them in to Matrix, including the possibility of other treatments being recommended or contributing to future patient benefit.

Oncologists also sought to downplay the importance of the trial to treatment, as this clinician explained:

> So one is when you see a patient initially … we don't really go into much detail of what SMP involves 'cos when they come to see … the complexity of the treatment … is vast and we perhaps don't have … all the results to make their initial treatment decision. So we'll go through about four, five scenarios and by that stage, you know, they're absolutely … saturated. So, you'll mention the Matrix, saying, 'Oh, and by the way, we're doing this study which doesn't involve anything else apart from blood tests. It's looking for a potential treatment in the future … you may or may not be eligible for it.' So, it's a sort of loose conversation and then they obviously meet with [the research nurse] who has a more detailed conversation about it.

But the way ... at the initial diagnosis we mention it as ... almost like an afterthought so it's not ... a focus 'cos it's not a first line treatment so it's not the focus of that. And then most patients actually don't really remember it ... it's only when ... they unfortunately relapse or ... we then go back to them and ... someone will say, 'Oh, oh, did the results come back from SMP2?' And then the majority of time we say, 'Actually, they have and you're not eligible' or they've failed, and then we have that dilemma about do you then re-biopsy them?

Making the pre-screen study and trial valuable to patients was therefore an ongoing process, a question of timing when to give information, as well as adjusting the amount and type of information being provided to the patient's circumstances. By offering more established kinds of personalised care as part of the recruitment process, the personalising impetus of genomic medicine in the process is reworked within caring practices. This also involved having to manage disappointment and make further decisions about trying again to see if the patients could be recruited. We observed discussions and were given examples of patients whose samples had been reanalysed several times in a concerted effort to get them on to the trial at a point at which 'time is running out'.

On other occasions where results from SMP2 were not expected to lead to involvement in the trial by clinicians but patients were nevertheless hopeful, practitioners sought to manage this, including via 'avoidance tactics' without 'dampen[ing] hope'. For example, nurses spoke with us about avoiding walking through a waiting area so as not to encounter a patient who had been calling every day for results.

Cultivating a sense among patients that the benefits of participation were greater than their own individual benefit was another strategy for managing potential disappointment, in the words of the senior CTA:

Most of the patients will enter strat med [Stratified Medicine Programme 2] with the understanding that it's going to help somebody else ... a lot of the patients don't care if it helps them. They just care that it helps somebody else. I've had patients say, 'As long as I don't have to go through the same thing that I'm go – you know, somebody else doesn't have to go through what I'm going through, then I'll sign up to anything.'

And why do you – why do you think that – that is?

I think they feel like they can give back, I think like they're giving some value. Their life is like some kind of a value, their experiences have given value to … research and to patients in the future. I think they want to see … especially lung cancer cured, yeah.

Invoking benefits for future patients, rather than the patient in the pre-screening study who was not able to make it on to the trial, was a way of offering a sense of purpose and contribution for patients with few treatment options and foreshortened futures. Consultants also prioritised other opportunities such as immuno-therapy (approved by NICE in 2017) where they viewed these options as more likely to prolong survival time. The trial therefore slotted into an ongoing process of managing patients' hopes and optimising their chances by prioritising treatments and keeping other options in reserve according to the patients' state of health and cancer type/results – as well as their capacity to cope with this information and decisions.

'Living in hope' (CTA) about the potential of the pre-screening study and trial involved difficult and painstaking work to try to optimise the prospects of a successful result by caring for the tissue itself. This included the CTA stewarding and tracking tissue as it moved between local laboratories (for sample preparation and then DNA extraction) and onwards to the national laboratory, as well as chasing results. It was also evident during biopsy procedures and laboratory analysis as practitioners sought to extract value and optimise the patient's chances of participation in a treatment arm of the trial. This was difficult and painstaking work given that the tissue sample being used for analysis was often very small, which meant that procuring and extracting DNA was a complex process resulting in a number of test failures. In order to offset the potential for failure, pathologists as well as geneticists and clinical trials staff described 'maximising the tissue' as well as thinking ahead to what might be needed from the tissue in the future (Swallow et al. 2020).

Making the screening study and trial work as a package inevitably involved tensions between staff as they sought to balance the different priorities of treatment and research. This is further illustrated in the extract from a fieldnote below, where the CTA is trying to find patients to consent to SMP2:

Each week the CTA double checks with each consultant whether she can recruit the patients she's identified as being suitable for SMP2. She checks with the consultant who seems reluctant to discuss 'I thought the Matrix had finished' 'it's not you again' ... It transpired that three of this consultant's patients wouldn't be suitable – the consultant describes these patients as 'knackered' and the CTA explains that she's not sure whether she believes him [this is the same consultant she feels doesn't understand the meaning or utility of SMP2/Matrix for lung cancer patients]. One of the patients had dementia and so couldn't be approached. The CTA checked with a different consultant whether she could consent the final 2 patients and following what was quite a lengthy discussion [I waited in the corridor] CTA explained to me that she would approach one of the patients ...

As I was stood chatting with both the CTA and a research nurse, a patient and their family member/friend headed to the consultant's room [consultant who is reluctant to allow CTA to recruit his patients] and the CTA smiles and whispers '[The consultant] smiled when he went past, did you see – he must have been the knackered patient, I didn't believe him at first!' Responding to this the research nurse asks 'is he ... being obstructive?' The CTA agrees and tells us how slow it's been for recruitment lately although also she stresses her efficiency, 'I've consented everyone!'

In an earlier observation the issue of numbers and progress with the trial also came up:

I asked whether she could show me the report that she sends each month to CRUK. The CTA explained that at the moment her 'numbers are really bad' and stresses that this will look like she's 'not performing' when actually 'it's not my fault' – 'I have my numbers of the year but it doesn't look like that.' I asked what happens if she doesn't get her quota of patients consented each month 'I don't know, I probably get called in to an office somewhere' – hesitant when I asked this question and kept reiterating that she'd consented enough patients for the year 'just keep on going' – showed January's numbers – 'look I consented 16 patients in this month'.

We got chatting about the observations we're doing in the labs – 'oh you can tell us why samples aren't being processed then – why they're just left ... you can spy for us' (laughs).

Here we can draw further insights into the work that key personnel such as CTAs do to try to make the pre-screening study and the trial work, persistently cajoling consultants, chivvying laboratories, recruiting allies such as our researcher, in an effort to meet recruitment targets. These excerpts also illustrate the concerns of staff who acquired an unwelcome sense of responsibility for the trial's slow progress, trying to recuperate its value by focusing on recruitment to the larger screening study instead – a study which also aims to transform the NHS's capabilities in genomic sequencing.

In this section we have explored how practitioners sought to make the pre-screening study and trial work for patients, and for the network and trial coordinators, via an array of calibration, articulation and uncertainty work. Deriving value from the trial for individual patients, the research programme and future patients was difficult and could be secondary to efforts to care for patients in the here and now. Nevertheless, practitioners expended considerable energy on trying to get a result of value that would offer patients access to the trial and further targeted treatments, including retesting, tracking samples and encouraging other practitioners to join these efforts. Calibrating patients' expectations was also an ongoing process of optimisation to offer sufficient but not excessive hope.

Patients accessing and being on trial

The complexities and attrition rate of the pre-screening study and trial, together with the poor health of patients and the pressures on the clinical team, also meant that we found it difficult to observe and interview patients through their journey from the pre-screening study to the trial. We only managed to interview a small number of patients on the trial, as well as another group of patients on the screening study who did not manage to get on to the trial. We approached recruitment with caution, aware of the precarious position of patients, the likelihood of deterioration, and difficulties with biopsy procedures and attrition. We were concerned not to add to the burden of work and engagement that the trial required from patients as well as healthcare staff.

As discussed above, part of the way in which practitioners sought to manage patients' expectations of the pre-screening study and trial was to provide specific details about their options at the optimum time so as not to 'saturate' patients with information or raise false hopes. They also sought to offer the opportunity of the trial at the right time when other options had been explored and exhausted. This meant that the patients we interviewed and observed when they were being recruited to SMP2 were often not told about Matrix explicitly. This was partly because of known problems with tissue analysis and the likelihood that no actionable mutations would be found, but it was also because some of these patients were very unwell and unlikely to survive to receive the results.

In observations and interviews with patients who consented to be part of SMP2, expectations of personalised treatments arising were nevertheless present, albeit in quite vague terms. An example was Richard, a man in his forties with advanced NSC lung cancer that was responsive to the ALK inhibitor, crizotinib. For Richard, surgery was not an option due to the spread of cancer to lymph areas and blood vessels. Personalised treatments were the very best the NHS had to offer and he wanted to play his part in their efforts to help him by being positive about his prospects:

> But I believe that that's an informed decision ... other people have done that for me ... we have this amazing system in this country ... if they've gone away and done these tests then I believe them. People make mistakes in all walks of life, I would, I would understand that if, if something went wrong ... at least you gave it a go and ... we're not ... saying, well that's the end of that then ... I'm a fighter and I'd like to think everybody's doing their very best ... to help me ...
>
> ... they've said, 'right okay, this is targeted, this is what we think is the best plan of option for you, and if it doesn't work, we gave it go and we'll try something else. And if that doesn't work, we'll try something else.' So ... why would I close any of those doors?
>
> I remember ... [my oncologist] ... telling me about these genetic mutations and that I was only a one in twenty case, and I actually had to say to him, 'sorry, is this a good thing or is this a bad thing?'... I think I've been taking these tablets for about eleven weeks now ... and they were talking about maybe a nine-month process ... I have good days, some days I have bad days, some days ... while I've got everyone, my family and professionals around me, while I've got everybody doing everything that they can, well, you stay positive don't you? ...

As well as keeping his future open, Richard also framed being part of research and experimentation, and trusting in clinicians, as part of progress towards a cure for future patients:

> people have said to me, 'oh it's a good job you didn't have this twenty years ago' ... Well maybe in twenty years' time, they'll be saying to people, well thank god we've got a cure for cancer now, because if this had happened to you twenty years ago, you'd be in this, all this experimental stage where no one really was a hundred per cent sure.

For Richard, helping himself with more personalised treatments was also about helping other patients to access this kind of medicine in the future, as he explained earlier in the interview: 'if I can be involved in that for my particular problems ... not just for me ... then why would I, why would I rebuff that opportunity ... I think that would be silly'.

This balancing act between personal and collective futures was also evident in an interview with another patient, Michael, who told us that he stopped smoking instantly after his diagnosis because 'you [health service] help me and I'll help myself' is his 'motto', and how he tried to get his mother to stop too. He went on to reflect on how being on the trial was helpful:

> It helps ... the tablet, it helps your own mind. That's it. But basically, you're helping other people behind you. 'Cause then ... my trial might say right, it works with their DNA. And then another part of it, that one, put the two of them together ... Bang. We've cured him ... I might go in ... a fortnight and she'll go, that tablet is working. It's no[t] growing. And it's no[t] breaking up. Take this other one. We've trialled it with other people ... Put the two tablets together and it might shrink and disappear.

Through these kinds of accounts, patients established their sense of purpose and hope, bolstering their identity as a worthwhile, active and valuable person as a way of coping with what was often a shocking discovery of cancer which encroached on their future (Chattoo and Ahmad 2003; Hubbard et al. 2010; Brown and de Graaf 2013).

Although lung cancer patients are typically less active in self-advocacy than other kinds of cancer patients, active engagement and self-advocacy was at times a strong feature of patients' and family members' accounts of Matrix in online lung cancer patient forums.

This included examples of patients encouraging each other to ask about Matrix, seek second opinions concerning eligibility and to chase results with the hospital. For example, in a discussion about the unpleasantness of the bronchoscopy to obtain a biopsy and the difficulties with waiting on results one patient commented:

> we were told about a month ago that they were asking [the hospital] for my biopsy. only now told that they had mislaid it. we kept having to ring the [hospital] just to warn others that if they haven't heard for a bit make sure that they haven't lost you in the system.[15]

Patients and relatives supported and advised each other about how to get on to the trial too, for example:

> First thing ask to take part in the National lung matrix, ours is in the [hospital] ask to be tested for EGFR its the cancer gene that determines whether they can use a non chemo drug such as immunotherapy. If your hospital doesn't do trials like ours … get a consultant at one that does. It sounds like you can't opt for radiotherapy if it has spread but everyone is different and how well you are.
>
> Don't take one person's expert opinion do your own research and both decide. If we had my wife would have been in a hospice by now and I have no doubt about that, now she has been in the garden all day and gone out shopping amazing difference in hospitals, and this isn't private our good old NHS.
>
> You are at the worse stage as you don't have enough info, like Brexit really, it gets better. The [hospital] is outstanding and I hear the [other hospital] is as good. Our Professor … is so passionate and yet the first thing the oncologist in [another hospital] said at diagnosis do you want some morphine to take home. Keep strong and keep positive

As this excerpt illustrates, patients expressed both gratitude and frustration with the NHS as part of these accounts, simultaneously evoking personal responsibility while also signalling commitment to a public spirit of care. Their accounts demonstrate the unevenness of information provision about the trial and about the capacity to access it. This mixing of emotions and values was a feature of what patients described as having 'nothing to lose' and a sense of taking control over advanced cancer through this kind of activity:

> you can only but ask (OR SHOUT) if you think you might be right for this. If you don't ask you don't get.

–

[name], just go for that link from [name] & see what happens.

COME ON SUNSHINE GO FOR IT !!!!!

Frustrations, typically focused on the NHS, ranged from difficulties with accessing the trial to waiting for results, as in the extracts below:

> Had 10 week break should get results tomorrow of the matrix trial, hopefully I might get lucky and get on a trial this time

> Having not qualified three times for new treatments so far. Don't get me wrong I am very happy for those who have the protein to be accepted, but from what I can see that is only a minority, even though I am told that they work just as well for the people who haven't got the protein but maybe not for so long, so to me in a word to me it is nothing short of rationing.

Through these kinds of exchanges forum contributors articulated their sense of individual and collective self-worth, resisting unwelcome kinds of stratification while advocating personalisation in other respects, framing the work of being a cancer patient or relative in this world of experimental medicine as one of persistence against the odds to try to get to the next level of access to treatment:

> My brother was signed up for SMP2, leading on to the Lung Matrix Trial, but his original biopsy returned a technical failure on the gene testing. It was simply too poor quality. They can't get another biopsy from his lung as his lung tumours are too small (the biggest is about 1.3cm) and although he has extensive brain mets, including one at 2.5cm, a biopsy of a brain met isn't standard NHS practice. Anyway, the good news is he might be ALK+ too, as a review of his original ALK test (initiated by the request for his biopsy block for SMP2) has been interpreted as having granular positivity for ALK. They can't confirm that without another biopsy, and they don't consider this as definitely ALK positive, but it's a ray of light. That review would never have come about if it wasn't for SMP2/Matrix. So, go for it … like [another forum user] I would say you never know what might come out of it!

'Rays of light' provide a sliver of hope for the future for these more active patients pursuing treatments, even as scientists and clinicians might have been much less optimistic. Although patients and relatives did engage with the molecular details of diagnosis as part of discussing their options, online exchanges were not places where lung cancer patients and relatives necessarily grouped around the details of specific subtypes. Instead they supported and encouraged each other, alongside family members, to move through the levels of access to acquire personalised information that might hold the promise of future therapies.

Other patients were less proactive in researching or engaging with detailed information, as was the case with the metastatic gynaecology patients encountering the VGT study as discussed in Chapter 3. Derek, a man in his sixties, had lung cancer which was diagnosed late and had spread to his spine. In an interview, he told us he too hoped for treatments from his participation in SMP2, something he described as 'selfish', but he also wanted to help future patients, such as his descendants. He was bewildered and shocked by his diagnosis and told us he coped with this by putting his trust in the clinicians, and not trying to find out too much about the details of his cancer. So his route into the study had been more passive than the kinds of approaches discussed above, as was the case with other patients we observed and interviewed. For these patients participation was part of their effort to 'carry on living as I did before', on the basis that something might come out of their participation, given that targeting treatments is better than a 'blanket' approach which 'bombard[s] everybody exactly the same'. The SMP2 study, and the possibilities of targeted treatments, were but one part of a wider approach to living with cancer rather than a unique source of particular promise.

For patients who were successful in getting on to the trial the benefits could be self-evident, just as they were for patients such as Richard, already on targeted treatments and engaging with research in SMP2. When asked directly about her reason for participating in the trial, another patient, Marion, who had recently had brain surgery because her cancer had spread, and had recently joined the trial, explained:

Well I don't see how it can hurt. Anything that's going to … that might have any kind of positive result has got to be good. It's better than doing nothing about it. And it might do something really positive.

And stop the cancer altogether. Because they can't guarantee that the brain tumour won't return again. Apparently, that's a possibility.

The possibility of stopping the cancer growing, which her husband, Malcolm, later described as 'arresting its development', drove Marion's involvement in the trial. As another patient in her forties, Victoria, noted, it 'buys you a bit more time'. Victoria was just finishing treatment as we interviewed her. She had previously recovered from ovarian cancer but had gone on to develop lung cancer. She explained,

Because obviously my cancer's not curable but it's treatable, but every time something stops working, we have to think, well what's the next thing, what is coming? I know there's lots and lots of research that's being done into lung cancer at the moment … how can you, how can you advance any sort of knowledge if you're not involved in, in trials really? And also, it does give you a good understanding of what the treatment landscape looks like, or might look like, and to me … it's helpful to know what things might be on horizon, or you know, what trials might be available …

Future-crafting of this sort involved the intensive and ongoing work of remaining hopeful. Janet recognised how treatments had improved since her sister had died from skin cancer several years previously. Janet was on the no-actionable genetic change (immunotherapy) arm of the trial (now in remission). She emphasised the importance of trust and fortitude:

You know, if it weren't for them, there'd be a hell of a lot of us not around still … so what do you do? You turn round and say, 'No I don't think I'll bother today,' so I could wake up and think, 'oh do you know what, I'll have a bit of cancer today'. So it's either put your trust in them and know that they can give you something what kills it or keeps it bay, or sit in a corner and slap your head against the wall. Fear worries me. Well sorry, I'm not that sort of person.

You know, just got to do what you've got to do, don't you, at the end of the day and you don't want to stop here, so you do it.

We interviewed Jenny, with her husband Paul, at a cancer centre. Both were in their seventies and Jenny had recently started a targeted treatment on one arm of the Matrix trial. They described how the Matrix trial (which Jenny transferred hospitals to join) had given them hope after Jenny had been told she was no longer responding to treatment. For Jenny and Paul this involved resisting the idea that she had only five months to live:

> [Paul] I've an issue with this because averages don't work. Anyway, so ... your response was, 'Give me anything.'
>
> [Jenny] Yeah, anything and everything (laughs) ... I'm really pleased to be on the trial and I think I'm very lucky because of what the consultant said right at the beginning, because the first thing I did was count the five months ... I think I really appreciate the trials because I think if it wasn't for them, if I believed what that ... consultant told me, I wouldn't be here. So I really think it is the trials that have helped.

Being on trial was often a last hope for patients, but it also offered reassurance and care, in part because it signalled that consultants were working hard to keep up with her cancer:

> [Jenny] Oh, they were absolutely fine. I mean they did say, they told me that it was affecting my liver ... and that there would be alternative treatment.
>
> [Paul] They were very positive about...
>
> [Jenny] They were, yeah.
>
> [Paul] ... that there's always something else. And they also ... said, 'There is another trial.' They'd already spoken (laughs softly) to [this hospital] and there's a trial now called the, the Lung Matrix Trial, which tries to pinpoint people with similar DNA or whatever. And ... she would go on that. So we were...
>
> [Jenny] Really positive then.
>
> [Paul] ... told, given bad news and then good news. So that was ... really good because it was ongoing. They also rang you later (laughs softly) didn't they...
>
> [Jenny] Yeah.
>
> [Paul] And said, 'If anything goes wrong, ring us. We may have another treatment for you here.'
>
> **Wow.**
>
> [Paul] Yeah. So I mean that side of it's been fabulous.
>
> [Jenny] Yeah, yeah.

[Paul] The only issue is they don't communicate very well (laughs softly) with each other, do they? Well this is it with hospitals. I don't think they do, do they?

The work of the hospitals to keep options open was a source of reassurance and hope. Jenny and Paul continued,

[Paul] [They told us] 'If that doesn't work, we'll ... have something else here.'

[Jenny] 'We'll, we'll always have something else for you.'

[...]

[Jenny] And that was a phone call to my house, you know, after I'd been, finished with [that hospital] ... I thought that was amazing, you know. So I thought, well if this doesn't work, maybe I can give them a ring...

Although these accounts contain familiar logics of promise and hope from trials which can also be found in patients' accounts of other sorts of trials and treatment, they also reference the promise of adaptability and responsiveness to cancer according to personal and specific genomic changes – key distinguishing features of this new generation of trials and the personalisation of treatment on offer.

For Janet, Jenny and Paul, personalisation via the trial also offered a more precise hope. Janet, even though she was on the non-actionable arm of the trial (i.e. her treatment was not based on genetic changes), nevertheless experienced the treatment as personalised:

when they did the second [biopsy] and they said they've actually got whatever it was they were looking for, I thought 'yes ... they've found something, they have found it' ... I think what must have gone through my head at the time was, well if they find whatever they're looking for in this DNA and they ... made ... some sort of drug or whatever the case may be ... I'd expect them to sort of like say to me, 'right we've done this, we've got this. This is what it is. It's from your DNA, it's from your body, so we know your body's going to accept this drug and it's going to help.'

I mean, it'll never go, I don't suppose. It'll never ever go, but the one on my lung has shrunk because ... I've had radiotherapy ... These in my neck ... I can't even feel them now, but like I say, if it weren't for ... all these drugs and putting stuff together and seeing what makes this ... do this, then I probably wouldn't be here.

For Jenny and Paul,

> [Paul] … being on a trial, there's always a risk of it not suiting you or it being cancelled because it suits you but it doesn't suit a lot of other people.
>
> […]
>
> [Paul] I think the Matrix way is better because it's trying to aim at suiting you, or you and a small percentage of people, and say 'for these people it's great, so we'll carry on; for these other people, it's not so good, so we'll do something else'. And I think that's the whole, that's –
>
> [Jenny] It's a lot more choice in treatments.

As Paul explained, this was more positive than his mother's experiences of undergoing chemotherapy:

> [Paul] [going on the trial] that was a big relief to both of us, actually, because … although you said … you'd spend a fortune on wigs, you didn't really want to, did you?
>
> [Jenny] (laughs) And said, if I had to wear a wig, I would have a lot of them (laughs) and very expensive (laughs).
>
> […]
>
> [Paul] Well, historically, I know … my mother died of cancer and had the most terrible chemotherapy, because it was just the same, they stuffed the same poisons into her as they did to everybody else … whichever cancer it was … And I think, nowadays, what they're doing is it's the same as going and getting a suit made to measure rather than buying one off the peg. It's … better for you and it might only be a tiny tweak.

As Jenny noted elsewhere, the totemic value of the trial brought an enhanced sense of personalisation: 'I got in my head that if they actually found some sort of treatment [that] shrunk mine … I should be offered it 'cause at the end of the day, it's part of me. You know, it's part of my body, it's my DNA.'

Maintaining hope while on the trial was, however, a complex affair that involved numerous balancing acts. As Paul noted, more time had to mean quality time: 'Well I think anything that holds out the possibility that she could have longer and better quality of life, I think these two things, longer, but we don't want longer if

there's not quality … So it's longer and better quality.' Patients on
the trial also described hoping to keep the 'cancer at bay' in Janet's
words, while also keeping open the possibility of a longer-term and
more remarkable result, as described by Michael:

> 'Cause that's what the tablet's to do. Just … it's to stop it growing
> and stop it spreading, breaking up and spreading. And if that happens
> it just means then you get on with your life…
>   … it's just something that's there and it's not going anywhere.
> That's it. So then maybe such-and-such'll get something that'll make
> it disappear altogether. But at least it's no[t] growing.

Other participants experimented with the hope that practitioners
are going to produce a 'magic cure', as Marion's husband Michael
put it. For example, in Victoria's interview she joked:

> What I told my consultant when I started it, I said, I want nothing
> less than a headline out of this, and she said, 'we'd go *Daily Mail*,'
> so it was a new and unexpected life goal (laughs). So yeah, no …
> peer review journals for it, cause we were going straight, straight for
> the top (laughs).

Here Victoria reflects on building rapport with clinicians and leaving
a legacy, thereby maintaining hope. As Michael explained this could
also involve avoiding certain trains of thought: 'I don't ask them
how long have I got … I'll know myself. So … but I just hope the
trial maybe worked for me and I get … I don't know if I've got two
weeks, two years or twenty years…'

However, in other respects, patients reflected on the need to lower
expectations (Gardner et al. 2015), as Victoria explained:

> I think also, as patients, there's got to be some sort of acceptance, so
> I suppose of the limits of what medicine can do … of course you
> want research to always be, pushing the boundaries … but in reality
> how does that translate into what can it actually do for you and does
> that mean that, you know, just because we can do something, well
> does that mean we should be keeping people alive at all costs … if I
> was going into my consultant every few weeks and saying … 'what
> are you doing to make sure that … you keep me alive, or you can
> cure my cancer?' we wouldn't be getting very far. We're having to
> work together to understand that we can't cure this, but we can …
> maintain my quality of life … and my health actually, you know, for
> as long as we possibly can.

Victoria's sense of partnership with the clinical team can, however, be contrasted with Janet's doubts about her care. Janet received treatment on the trial that was not funded by the NHS and she described her anxieties that in a year's time they might decide not to fund the treatment further. She raised these concerns with the consultant who said they would 'cross that bridge when we come to it', bracketing the future to protect patients from the possibility of failure and disappointment.

Being on the trial involved living with uncertain futures where much was at stake. It also involved managing side-effects and disappointments with care, as the extract below from one of the Cancer Patient Discussion forums illustrates:

> It's been many months since I have posted an update for the simple reason is the phase 2 drug trial (matrix Arm C) has been doing what it says on the tin ... keep the tumour growth at bay.
>
> Side effects ... feel very tired on the recovery week due to low red and white blood counts (3 weeks of drug and 1 week off for recovery) and cough gets worse near the end of each cycle however apart from that all has been all good.
>
> Had 6 weekly CT scan just after xmas and they saw very slight growth of the tumour, plus a small secondary bone cancer (treated with radiotherapy) so 'we' started looking for a plan B which also included possibly moving my treatment [to another hospital].
>
> The CT scan last week – the trial drugs have completely failed, or has the cancer mutated so the drugs are no longer effective? Noticeable tumour growth plus fluid on lung, second lymph node has growth to a possible infected size. Probable infection in liver.
>
> All a bit of a shock as we had our rose-tinted glasses on and were hoping just small amount of small growth.
>
> Well shit happens and we move on. We always knew that I would have to be off any treatment before moving onto another trial assuming something is available. We are just off the current trial a bit earlier than expected.
>
> Bring on the next trial...[16]

Here we see the work of reinterpreting failure and orienting to the future, as well as some of the problems associated with too much hope being attached to these trials by patients and family members. Patients nevertheless welcomed the care they had received while on the trial, particularly the time spent with research nurses discussing difficulties around treatment and uncertainties. For Marion and Michael the trial also provided them with the opportunity to feel more involved in their care, affording an extra level of care: 'giving me an MOT', in Michael's words, and, for Marion, feeling 'very closely monitored ... that makes me feel good ... it's better than just leaving you not knowing what's happening'. Victoria also welcomed this:

> so I'd rather, in a way that they were taking a bit of care of me rather than sending me away, see you in six months and see if your arm's dropped off or anything ... I tell all of my friends it's like going up another level in a computer game ... Do not go to level one, go straight up the lift to level three, where five nurses are waiting for you. So yes, it's lovely, I feel much more looked after.

The importance of developing relationships and spending time with healthcare staff was also important as Jenny and Paul described:

> [Paul] And it is that sort of positive from some of the nurses. We had a lovely nurse, [name of nurse], in, in [hospital] who used to tell us all about what she was doing and where she'd been.
>
> [Jenny] Yeah, everybody's got...
>
> [Paul] And the girls up here in the—
>
> [Jenny] ... time, time to talk to you.
>
> [Paul] Yeah.
>
> [Jenny] You know, it's not as though you're a – I don't know. 'Sit there and we haven't time cos we're busy.'
>
> [Paul] Yeah.
>
> [Jenny] You know, everybody has the time to sit down and have a chat with you.
>
> [Paul] But ... here ... the nurses and the, the consultants always seem to have a decent time to spend with you.
>
> [Jenny] Yeah, yeah, there's no rush. There really isn't.
>
> [Paul] I've never felt rushed out of the consultancy...
>
> [Jenny] No.
>
> [Paul] ... without being asked if there was anything else we wanted to talk about.

[...]

I think that's it really. We just feel that there's caring people, with time.

As this exchange illustrates, being on the trial meant spending time and developing partnerships with clinicians which was experienced as comforting; an example of how trials create the space for additional carework from busy staff, which patients and relatives greatly value.

For patients facing an advanced lung cancer diagnosis, adaptive trials such as Matrix are an opportunity to extend severely diminished futures, keeping options open and being positive about living with cancer even though there is no cure. This was articulated in terms of being fortunate to be part of something advanced or cutting-edge in some cases, and via a detailed engagement with the particularities of research design or experimental treatments in other situations (particularly in the online forums), with the idea of tailored or targeted treatments resonating with commonsense understandings that precision is better than blanket or one-size-fits-all approaches. For some of these, often younger patients and their relatives, advocating for participation in trials and engaging in detail with the processes and its complexities as they tried to negotiate access to experimental treatments was a way of optimising their health despite the cancer diagnosis, somewhat mirroring the work of nurses chasing samples and results. For other patients their engagement with the trial and pre-screening study was more passive, a matter of trusting in the clinicians in an effort to gain more time, particularly for older patients, as was also the case among the gynaecological cancer patients discussed in the previous chapter. Persistence, fortitude and positivity were nevertheless key virtues for patients across these different groups.

Participation in the pre-screening study and trial was also, on occasion, an opportunity to demonstrate commitment to helping other patients in the future, although this was inevitably framed as a secondary benefit in favour of personal benefits. Accessing more personalised care was another valuable part of participation; spending time with nursing staff was particularly important for patients as they sought to carry on with their lives and maintain self-worth in the face of narrowing horizons. Participation could nevertheless generate uncertainties and anxieties about waiting, about treatments after the trial or side-effects and lack of effectiveness of treatments. As with the breast and gynaecological cancer patients discussed in the previous chapters, adaptive trials generate promise and hope for the future among lung cancer patients, but this can be fleeting, contingent and overshadowed by ongoing and growing uncertainties and worsening health.

Conclusion

Adaptive trials are a key feature of the personalised cancer medicine landscape, offering patients experimental, targeted treatments and reconfiguring institutional arrangements to mainstream next-generation sequencing as part of care. In the case of lung cancer patients, this offers a new set of options for patients with some of the worst outcomes, given that lung cancer tends to be diagnosed at an advanced stage. Patients affected with lung cancer also tend to have less financial and social capital with which to manage their condition, since it is associated with disadvantage. Practitioners are therefore keen to make these new opportunities work for these patients, but they are also operating in difficult circumstances, in services where resources are pressurised and outcomes are disappointing. The screening and trial arrangements of which they are a part are also complex and difficult to implement, not least because obtaining and analysing a sample of sufficient quality involves many intricate steps and numerous actors, taking time and asking patients to wait when their futures are already foreshortened and their health continues to deteriorate. Making this trial work – for institutions and for patients – therefore took considerable care, marked by calibration, articulation and navigation work for practitioners and, at times, patients and their relatives.

Such work always has to be weighed against the perceived needs of patients for whom care in the moment can trump the possibility of future treatments emerging from the trial. Practitioners and patients sought to maintain hope and salvage other kinds of value, such as care in the moment, when results were disappointing. Participation or engagement with the trial and its possibilities could generate additional uncertainties, anxieties and disappointments that also had to be managed by staff, patients and families. Patients did this work alongside their relatives, sometimes in public forums where they engaged in detail with the trial arrangements and processes. But for other patients there was less engagement with the technicalities of the trial and more of a focus on relations of trust and care with clinicians – two different ways of enacting hope with persistence, fortitude and positivity. Together, these activities and expectations formed part of an ongoing process of optimising the possibility of the trial that worked alongside efforts to optimise treatments and sequencing infrastructures to deliver the new era of personalised cancer medicine.

In her study of adaptive trial methodologies, Montgomery notes that

> the temporal politics of adaptive design straddle a ... diffuse set of scientific institutions, from profit-seeking big Pharma to publicly- and philanthropically-funded academia. What is at stake is not so much the creation of commercial value through the promise of a given vision, but the creation of value – moral, epistemic and commercial – through the ability to know the unknowns and to fix the future as it unfolds. (2017a: 237)

We can see these forms of value emerge, diverge and fade across the different levels at which the trial and pre-screen study on which it depended were orchestrated and experienced by practitioners and patients. Making a success of the trial for practitioners and for patients could mean different things, but in each case it involved ongoing processes of careful tinkering in an effort to chase and realise value, even when this could be fleeting or minimal. This work kept the trial going, enabling the extraction of other kinds of commercial value in the future through drug development and improved trial processes. Big pharma was remote from the clinic, but the hopes inspired by the possibility of 'drugs that work' for current and future patients were ever present. Yet practitioners, relatives and patients trying to make the pre-screening study and the trial deliver personalised care to patients also generated value for the consortia, institutions, funders and investors in this new form of personalised medicine. This spurred further faith and investment in the UK bioeconomy, enhancing scale, and innovating new kinds of pathways, research consortia, valuation practices, gene panels and, of course, the data required for the innovation of new drugs. As we go on to discuss in the next chapter on whole genome sequencing studies, these processes of generation and extraction of data are crucial to the promise of personalised cancer medicine, even if it is not yet being delivered at scale to current patients.

Notes

1 www.cancerresearchUK.org/funding-for-researchers/how-we-deliver-research/our-research-partnerships/stratified-medicine-programme (accessed 10 July 2019).
2 www.ecmcnetwork.org.UK/national-lung-matrix-trial (accessed 8 July 2019).
3 www.birmingham.ac.UK/research/activity/mds/trials/crctu/trials/lung-matrix/index.aspx (accessed 8 July 2019).
4 www.ecmcnetwork.org.UK/news/announcement/national-lung-matrix-trial-update-birmingham-ctu (accessed 8 July 2019).
5 www.birmingham.ac.UK/research/activity/mds/trials/crctu/trials/lung-matrix/professionals/design-treatments.aspx (accessed 9 July 2019).
6 www.ecmcnetwork.org.UK/news/announcement/over-1800-lung-cancer-patients-screened-through-stratified-medicine-initiative (accessed 8 July 2019).
7 www.ecmcnetwork.org.UK/news/announcement/stratified-medicine-programme-phase-2-update (accessed 8 July 2019).
8 www.ecmcnetwork.org.UK/news/announcement/smp2-and-nlmt-programme-updates (accessed 8 July 2019).
9 www.ecmcnetwork.org.UK/news/announcement/smp2-and-nlmt-network-2017-review (accessed 8 July 2019).
10 www.birmingham.ac.UK/research/activity/mds/trials/crctu/trials/lung-matrix/patients-public/get-involved.aspx (accessed 8 July 2019).
11 www.birmingham.ac.UK/research/activity/mds/trials/crctu/trials/lung-matrix/professionals/recruitment.aspx (accessed 8 July 2019).
12 www.birmingham.ac.UK/research/activity/mds/trials/crctu/trials/lung-matrix/participating-sites/index.aspx (accessed 8 July 2019).
13 https://twitter.com/BHPComms/status/1032654129687154689 (accessed 8 July 2019).

14 www.cancerresearchUK.org/about-us/cancer-news/press-release/2018-11-20-mirati-therapeutics-joins-cancer-research-UKs-stratified-medicine-programme (accessed 20 June 2020).

15 https://community.macmillan.org.UK/cancer_types/lung-cancer/f/lung-cancer-forum/93278/lung-matrix-trial—experiences?Page=0#772820 (accessed 20 June 2020).

16 https://community.macmillan.org.UK/cancer_types/lung-cancer/f/lung-cancer-forum/123798/its-all-gone-a-bit-pete-tong (accessed 20 June 2020).

5

Genomics at scale: participation to build the bioeconomy

Genomic research, with the aim of developing personalised cancer therapies, is not just being pursued through trials or smaller-scale studies in cancer clinics and laboratories. It is increasingly taking place on larger, national and industrial scales too, as data is gathered *en masse* from patients and publics (Hilgartner 2017). In this chapter we investigate one such flagship national genomic sequencing programme to explore how genomic data, alongside other health and social data, is being gathered via mainstream healthcare services and shared with companies so that its value can be rendered into new molecular profiling technologies and targeted drugs. Focusing on Genomics England's 100,000 Genomes Project, we trace the ways in which data-rich healthcare futures are being crafted via cancer patients' and professionals' engagements with whole genome sequencing (WGS), exploring how participants' everyday experiences sit within a wider nexus of complex relationships and rearrangements of the NHS. Throughout we trace the kinds of futures articulated and mobilised by 'the genomics vanguard' (Hilgartner 2017: 27) of politicians and policymakers, together with the experiences of practitioners and patients, contrasting bigger promissory futures with the range of contingent, sometimes doubtful, at other times quietly hopeful futures crafted by patients and practitioners involved in making this initiative happen on the ground.

We could tell the story of the development of these initiatives through familiar framings of innovation, focusing on the rapidly advancing capacity and reduced costs of DNA sequencing and information technology as the main driver of progress. But to do so would be to miss some of the crucial political, economic and organisational changes in how data, institutions and value are being reconfigured to enable and extend these initiatives, changes which official discourses of success tend not to register. As Hilgartner has argued, to understand how technoscience such as genomic sequencing is a vehicle for the transformation of mainstream healthcare, we need to engage with the political and economic processes at stake, or in Hilgartner's words, 'how institutions, discourses, identities, constitutions, and imaginaries shape modes of decision making and guide public reason' (2017: 6). This includes tracing the production and effects of promissory and official discourses that underpin these developments: the futures envisaged for patients, services and the nation, the measures and processes underpinning governance and successful implementation, and the personal stories and affective repertoires of practitioners, advocates and participants. Considering what kinds of value are created for whom through these processes, and the work this involves for particular actors, is also key to our analysis, including with respect to how it is revealed or obscured in practice, replicating or subverting the roles ascribed to key actors through official discourses.

We interviewed a range of practitioners involved with the project at one institution which was part of a regional consortium – four of the project leads, the three nurses involved, and clinicians and scientists involved in implementation (including nurse consultants, histopathologists, pathologists, geneticists, oncologists, clinical scientists and biomedical scientists). We also observed 16 consenting clinic sessions (sometimes with two or three patient appointments) and interviewed 17 patients and three family members about their experiences of taking part in the project after these consent meetings. Interviews and observations were carried out between 2016 and 2018. We spoke to patients affected by breast, colorectal, gynaecological, brain and blood cancers. Participants ranged in age from the forties to the eighties. Some of these patients were in the early stages of breast cancer, prior to treatment, others were in remission following surgery for colorectal cancer, and some had more advanced or recurrent breast, brain or gynaecological cancers or were on long-term maintenance treatments for blood cancer.

In the next section, we trace how the promise of national genomic data and its analysis are articulated and realised as a form of economic growth and marketising public services, focusing on the 'knowledge-control regimes' (Hilgartner 2017: 13) of bioethics and the 'participatory turn', arguing that both are crucial to the realisation of biovalue from these large-scale programmes. This includes two important 'governing frames' (Hilgartner 2017: 13) which elaborate previous forms of participation – extending informed consent and public engagement/participation, including via evolving ideas and practices of 'genomic literacy'.

Genomics and the health of the nation

As Fortun wrote in his ethnography of the Icelandic genomics company deCODE's sequencing of the genomic assets of the Icelandic nation:

> Genomics is building new zones of intensities, places in and between the lab, the corporation, the experimental assemblage … the successful scientists and corporations will be those who can continually rearrange software, hardware, netware into hybrid combinations that create new intensities … Completion isn't promised by genomics, future becomings are. (Fortun 2008: 47)

A decade after these insights, we see the further intensification of value in a complex global network of market-data assemblages offering the promise of further growth in the bioeconomy. Companies set up by nation-states, such as Genomics England, commercial actors and state-based assets such as the NHS all operate in these zones. A great deal of attention is focused on commercial direct-to-consumer genomic tests. But the marketisation of genomic data is taking place through the auspices of public health providers such as the NHS as well. This involves key partnerships with commercial organisations involved in sequencing and analysing genomic and other NHS data in order to build capacity in the UK bioeconomy.

Since its establishment, Genomics England has developed complex governance arrangements to ensure that companies working with patients' genomic data are appropriately vetted, and that the data remains secure. Companies involved in this work become service providers, which might involve providing data and/or the interpretation of data or other technical services. These companies range in size and scale, but their international links to other national sequencing endeavours are clear. For example, Congenita, a spin-out company from the UK's Sanger Institute, funded by the Wellcome Trust, developed its clinical decision support software called Sapientia through involvement in Genomic England's 100,000 Genomes Project. In 2018 Congenita signed Memorandums of Understanding with Chinese companies and health providers at a trade event in China, which took place alongside a state visit by the then prime minister, Theresa May. These meetings received considerable press coverage in the run-up to Brexit as they became, for some, emblematic of the UK's capacity to develop global markets beyond the EU. The company's press release noted:

> Underlining Congenica's expansion and potential in China, it was one of only 5 UK companies to attend the signing event held in Beijing. Hosted by UK Secretary of State for International Trade, Dr Liam Fox, and China's ex-Vice Minister for NHFPC, Jin Xiaotao, each Government set out their vision for the future of digital health and confirmed the opportunities for international collaboration and trade.

The press release went on to give details of how the company had previously entered into an agreement to provide services for the Chinese '100K Wellness Pioneer Project', hosted by the Beijing 4P Health Research Institute. Congenica also has a contract with BGI Genomics in China and Series B fundraising to build its business, including investment from BGI.

The 100,000 Genomes Project emerges as more than just a project to provide UK patients with genomic information and the possibility of targeted drugs sometime in the future. It is also more than a matter of delivering sequencing and laboratory services differently in English hospitals: it is part of the development of the UK's commercial capacity, spun out by scientists who established their research with support from philanthropic and public funders committed to open genomic data, as UK businesses become embedded in a major new venture to transform the healthcare system through genomics.

The development of national genomic sequencing initiatives is not just driven by technological breakthroughs and reducing sequencing costs, as popular histories of genomics would have it. Instead this process was fundamentally enabled by a key set of political and institutional changes, led by state-actors and agencies and aimed at opening up population data and markets simultaneously. This is not so much a story of the 'invisible hand of the market' in Adam

Smith's famous formulation, as it is a story of the 'invisible hand of the state' (Goven and Pavone 2015). Monetising the nation's genomic assets is part of the marketisation of publicly funded health systems such as the NHS in post-austerity Britain (Hockings 2014).

This vision for genomic sequencing at scale, embedded across the health service, was largely 'top down' – what Hilgartner (2017: 27) calls a 'vanguard vision'. It was not broadly conceived within the scientific or medical community or the wider nation, but generated within elite scientific and government establishments. As Samuel and Farsides (2017) have written, the roots of what would become Genomics England can be traced to a House of Lords Science and Technology Committee report from 2009 (whose special advisor was Professor Tim Aitman, who would later become one of the leaders of the Scottish Genome Partnership), where the committee argued for 'a strategic vision for genomics in the UK'. The government set up the Human Genomics Strategy Group in response, chaired by Professor Sir John Bell, who would go on to sit as a non-executive director on the board of Genomics England. Bell also holds this position on the board of Roche (a prominent pharmaceutical and genomics sequencing company) as well as a host of other public and corporate appointments, including a period as president of the Academy of Medical Sciences (2006–11). The group's 2012 report, *Building on our inheritance: Genomic technology in healthcare*,[1] articulated the vision on which Genomics England would be based. Bell wrote in the Foreword:

> At present, we are in a position of strength. As the recent life sciences strategy highlighted, the UK is a recognised world leader in biomedical sciences and is home to many of the leading academic and commercial research centres spearheading the global development of genomic medicine and furthering the use of Clinical Genetics. This gives the UK an outstanding opportunity to exploit its scientific lead, via the NHS – a unique service delivery environment in which clinically validated genomic medicine will be able to thrive. The challenge is to make our vision a reality for the benefit of the NHS, for the benefit of the UK biomedical industry and, above all, for the benefit of patients and their families.
>
> It is also to move sufficiently rapidly that our leadership position is not undermined by other countries who have also recognised this opportunity and are now pursuing it. (Human Genomics Strategy Group 2012: 3–4)

The emphasis on leadership, nationhood, economic growth and the NHS as a valued public asset to be put to work to preserve its benefits for patients now and in the future has come to dominate the promissory discourses of this emergent field (Tarkkala et al. 2019). This gives a particularly British twist to the emphasis on genomics as a platform for global transformation, captured in a McKinsey Global Institute report of 2013 which called it one of 12 disruptive technologies that will 'transform life, business, and the global economy'.[2]

In the midst of a prolonged period of austerity in the UK, genomic research became a vehicle through which the British state, together with scientific and medical funding bodies and institutions, could transform the NHS to advance economic growth and social benefits in partnership with the private sector. Genomics England was set up as a state-owned company to coordinate and deliver these benefits, working in partnership with charitable funders and the private sector to sequence 100,000 genomes of cancer and rare disease patients by 2017. At a time when state funding to healthcare services was being reduced,[3] an initial £100 million of government funds was directed towards this flagship project aimed at transforming the NHS. This was part of a package of deals estimated to be worth £300 million, including a contract with the sequencing company Illumina (Sample 2014). The launch of the 100,000 Genomes Project was timed to coincide with the 65th anniversary of the NHS, and was given the personal backing of the then prime minister, David Cameron. Cameron focused on the transformation of the diagnosis and treatment of 'devastating diseases' in the NHS and beyond. Genomics England's press release at the time described the project as 'world leading research organisations join[ing] forces'.[4] The deal with Illumina was reported as being worth around £78 million for the company to deliver WGS, but it was also noted that Illumina would invest more than double this amount in this work in England, 'creating new knowledge and jobs in the field of genomic sequencing'. Alongside Illumina, the Wellcome Trust also invested a further £27 million in its Genome Campus in Cambridge where Genomics England's operations would be based, together with the Sanger Institute, one of the leading institutions involved in the Human Genome Project. This clustering of investments and location was further enhanced by Medical Research Council funding of £24 million to develop computing capacity and an NHS contribution of £20 million.

As well as building infrastructure, transforming healthcare and economic growth to position the UK at the forefront of the 'global race to implement genomic technology', it was noted that the expectation was that 'around 40,000 NHS patients could benefit directly from the research'. A transformed NHS was positioned as leading the way in contemporary healthcare through this initiative. The press release on the launch of Genomics England quotes Simon Stevens, NHS England's chief executive at the time:

> The NHS is now set to become one of the world's 'go-to' health services for the development of innovative genomic tests and patient treatments, building on our long track record as the nation that brought humanity antibiotics, vaccines, modern nursing, hip replacements, IVF, CT scanners and breakthrough discoveries from the circulation of blood to the existence of DNA.
>
> The NHS' comparative advantage in unlocking patient benefits from the new genomic revolution stems from our unique combination of a large and diverse population, with universal access to care, multi-year data that spans care settings, world-class medicine and science and an NHS funding system that enables upstream investment in prevention and new ways of working as demonstrated by this ground-breaking 100,000 Genomes Project.

In a session at the 2017 Bio International Convention, David Cameron, a prominent backer of the project, described his role in setting up the 100,000 Genomes Project as having been shaped by his experience of being a father to Ivan, his disabled son, who had a rare disease (and died at the age of 6 in 2009). He said that this had had a big influence on his thinking about science, discovery and life sciences, and was one of the reasons he commissioned the 100,000 Genomes Project and had the first sequenced genome delivered to his desk. Cameron said that he wanted to develop the life sciences and the wider economy through this project, reflecting that the NHS has the advantage of enormous amounts of usable data on which the project would draw.[5] He also referred to another feature of the discussions and politics around the NHS during his government, which focused on failings and reforms. Cameron had written about this in the tabloid newspaper *The Sun* one year before the official launch of the 100,000 Genomes Project. Additionally, in a report in *The Telegraph* his criticism was set out in emotive language of 'love' for the 'national treasure' that is the NHS, shaped by his experience of being a father to Ivan, yet contrasted with the need to deal with the problems of 'cover ups' and elderly care, and the need for medical advances in the NHS: 'We don't demonstrate that love by covering up things that go wrong. Or by pretending the NHS can just ignore the big challenges it faces.'

As a King's Fund report reviewing the NHS under the then coalition government (Ham et al. 2015) noted, Cameron and his government had a troubled relationship with this iconic British institution, spending much of their term of office developing, implementing and trying to repair the problems arising from the fraught Health and Social Care Act (2012) in the face of trenchant criticism from medical and patient communities. Cameron had to temper his focus on privatisation, service improvements and marketisation through this period, turning to focus on patient needs, for example through a commitment to keeping waiting times down.

The 100,000 Genomes Project was the ideal vehicle for transformation in this fraught context; a way of generating value by capitalising on the assets of the NHS, transforming the bioeconomy and healthcare for the twenty-first century. Its success hinged, above all, upon patients and their families participating in the venture, which, in turn, relied upon the trust and confidence of patients and the wider public. This would build on other large-scale projects, such as UK Biobank, and draw on the UK's global reputation for robust oversight via bodies such as the Human Genetics Commission. The Commission had, in fact, been disbanded in 2012 as part of a process of removing Whitehall 'quangos', so a new committee and oversight process had to be established as part of Genomic England's work. The close alignment of the project with NHS data and resources increased the perceived need for comprehensive and robust ethics, not least because of public controversy around the opt-out policies of the failed Care.Data initiative and deCODE Genomics Ltd. A series of public and professional consultation exercises underlined the importance of getting these processes right, given ongoing public concerns about insurance companies accessing data, the moratorium on this practice notwithstanding.

It was within this context that the then Chief Medical Officer (CMO) for England set up a group to provide advice on the ethical issues involved with the 100,000 Genomes Project, led by Professor

Mike Parker from Oxford University.[6] Informed consent was especially salient here, given the difficulties with past national projects such as that of Iceland, and the technical and organisational arrangements around this formed an important part of the group's work. The advisory group outlined what they called an 'appropriate and rational' approach to the ethical issues in a letter to the CMO in 2013. Stressing the guiding principles of decision making and commitments to the public interest, patients and the NHS, they placed considerable emphasis on the processes of informed consent and patient and public involvement and engagement. The group noted that data could not be irreversibly de-identified, so there was a need for data-access agreements and accountable governance processes that would 'provide participants, and the public, with the assurances they require and promote acceptability and involvement', especially since private companies would be involved in testing and possibly also other services. Again, the group stressed the importance of policies and procedures to ensure that commercialisation was in the public interest and of benefit to the NHS to ensure public confidence and participation.

These considerations formed the basis of the group's recommendations about informed consent processes, in which the importance of 'broad consent' that did not present too much of a burden to staff and patients was stressed. This involved considerable refinement and specification of what 'informed' should mean in this context. Although no doubt familiar with the extensive ethical and social scientific literature on how consent in many medical settings is not based on participants making dispassionate choices, but on a mixture of reasoning which depended on the context, including a sense of commitment to the health service and to the professionals involved in their direct care (Corrigan 2003; Dixon-Woods and Tarrant 2009), the committee had to use standard and established governance mechanisms to establish the credibility of the programme. This presented a number of challenges. A key issue was the difficulty of combining consent for data to be analysed as part of care and as part of research, both known and unknown. This blurred the line between care and research in a way that ethicists are often concerned to avoid because of the problem of 'therapeutic misconception', wherein patients consent because they are motivated by an expectation of improved care. This may leave them vulnerable to being misled or disappointed, rather than enabling a form of 'altruism' which ideally should determine their involvement in the logic of contemporary research ethics (Dheensa et al. 2018).

The importance of securing consent to future use of the data, which would drive the service transformation and economic benefits sought from the programme, was such that patients' opportunities to receive results became conditional on their consent for their data to be used in research. To avoid the need to go back to patients in the future about what precisely this research would involve, given that future uses cannot be known in advance, the group reasoned that a clear governance process for deciding on appropriate use and access would need to be put in place on participants' behalf, and recommended that this should be discussed in the consent process to give participants confidence to proceed. Moreover, they noted, 'participants will also need to understand that consenting to research involves a waiver of any personal rights to benefit from commercial exploitation. Mechanisms will need to be introduced to ensure that the NHS benefits where data from this programme are put to commercial use.' These recommendations narrowed the burden but also the boundaries of choice considerably – participants were given choices about what kinds of additional information they might want to receive, but were not invited to decide what kinds of research their samples or data could be used for. Here the possibilities for future research using the data accrued were deemed more valuable than the opportunities for individual crafting of involvement, the latter of which was seen as more of a potential burden than an opportunity.

Processes for developing and enacting these complex arrangements for informed consent constitute important governing frames in projects of this scale and complexity – they are as key to their realisation as sequencing technologies and laboratory standards. Yet informed consent processes are known to be problematic in practice, given to ritualised and superficial performances, what Corrigan (2003) aptly called 'empty ethics'. The committee therefore tried to make informed consent more meaningful by offering clarity and managing expectations. The group were particularly concerned with the question of how to report back information to patients in this emergent area of medical science, including how clinicians would be supported to make judgements and how families would be supported to manage the implications of results. The need for participants to make choices about data relevant to other family members had to be managed, as was the need for ongoing professional development and resources for re-contacting patients over time. These considerations point to one of the key challenges in this area: how to make results meaningful in the absence of clear and established protocols for interpretation, given the experimental nature of the science and the complexity of the data involved.

This is part of a new style of scientific governance that Braun et al. (2010) call 'reflexive governance', encompassing participation and engagement with a range of experts, including critical social scientists. Another important aspect of these forms of governance is participation by patients and publics, with a great deal of emphasis placed on inclusion and engagement. Education, support and training for staff and patients was particularly important. This extended engagement and cultivation of ethical participation (Braun et al. 2010) was seen as pivotal to the successful implementation of this part of the programme. A range of responsibilities for practitioners and patients to participate, learn and engage with new choices and forms of interpretation were therefore anticipated, in contrast to the circumscribed rights to choose how one's data might be capitalised, as discussed above. This framed additional responsibilities for a wider pool of potential participants from the public more generally, anticipating an expansion of participation in genomic research in the future. At the same time, the committee also prescribed a range of responsibilities for project leads and other practitioners involved in its delivery to take a role in education and public communication about the project, including about the relationship between the state and the market that is at its heart.

Genomics England took up these recommendations as part of its efforts to 'build a social contract' for the initiative,[7] and went on to establish a detailed informed consent and data governance process as well as a wide-ranging series of events, publications and a website with extensive resources for participants and links to training initiatives for staff. An ethics advisory group also became an established and important aspect of these governance arrangements. The consent form, initially lengthy and complex, went through a number of revisions and iterations as the project proceeded, partly in an effort to clarify and shorten sections to enable the process to be completed in less time. Genomics England has also sought to develop resources aimed at educating publics, professionals and participants about genomics, after identifying a lack of awareness about this area of science as part of a programme of improving 'genomic literacy'.[8] Here practitioners and publics acquire responsibilities for becoming more educated and educating others about genomics and its implications for health, in order that genomic medicine can be developed successfully. Notable among these initiatives is the 'Socialising the Genome' project, which includes a number of short YouTube videos utilising animation. One of these videos involves a play on the confusion between genomes and gnomes and features a cartoon gnome 'fishing' for pieces of DNA. This is prominently displayed on the Genomics England website and has been taken up in consent processes too.

The Genomics England website as a whole has more resources, case studies and patient testimonies concerning rare disease, as part of its efforts at engagement and education, reflecting the relative success of this part of the programme in terms of recruitment and delivery of results compared with those regarding cancer. For cancer patients there is, instead, a series of hedged statements about the ambition to deliver results in the future, and a lack of specificity about how and when this will happen, which contrasts with some of the earlier stated ambitions for the project. There is also a focus on explaining how the project has evolved and the technical difficulties that have been overcome in the process, for example the move from using formalin-fixed samples to fresh, frozen samples which are easier to analyse.

The website presents project news in relation to the numbers of genomes sequenced and features a counter to illustrate this. Numerical milestones are presented as important markers of success for the project. There is also considerable hype about the benefits of the programme, which sits at odds with the working groups' recommendations in this regard. For example, in a story about more than 70,000 sequences being completed on the 70th anniversary of the NHS, it was reported that Health Minister Lord O'Shaughnessy said:

> Genetic sequencing can revolutionise healthcare by offering truly personalised care to patients and their families. This project is a shining example of a partnership between the public sector, the life sciences industry and the research community – with NHS patients reaping the benefits. Genomic medicine is no longer a thing of the future, it's here now and helping to save lives.[9]

These kinds of promissory claims are more prominent than information about the involvement of commercial companies in the project,
which is scattered across the site and difficult to connect together
to form a picture of what kinds of roles these companies are taking,
and the financial arrangements involved.

   Together, these recommendations and practices constitute the
100,000 Genomes Project as a vehicle for the transformation of the
national economy and health service, monetising the genomic data
of the nation to change how medicine is delivered, and responsibilising
practitioners, patients and publics to become genomically literate
in order to deliver these benefits. To enable and enact this transformation, institutions, practitioners, publics and patients acquire new
responsibilities for participation, engagement and deliberation, but
these are carefully circumscribed within a web of governance and
educational arrangements which limit participant choices and, for
cancer patients in particular, have not delivered personalised information on the scale envisaged by some of the more optimistic accounts
of politicians and leading civil servants. The importance of not
burdening patients with too much information and too many choices
as part of the consent process can be contrasted with the emphasis
elsewhere on educating and informing patients about the programme
and the science involved as part of 'socialising the genome'. Presented
as short, fun encounters, these activities expose and seek to remedy
the deficit in public understanding about genomics through a growing
portfolio of educational tools and events, which produces an audience
with responsibilities to engage in turn. At the same time, however,
as we go on to consider later in this chapter, the details of the
economic arrangements at the heart of the programme or the choices
with regard to investment in personalised therapies versus other
kinds of structural public health interventions targeting the causes
of cancers are opaque and less easy to engage with and critique.

Transformations in cancer care: participation for practitioners

Transformative visions and the knowledge-control regimes that seek
to implement them are, of course, key features of how genomics at
scale took shape in the UK bioeconomy. But as Hilgartner (2017)
amply demonstrates in the case of the Human Genome Project,

vanguard visions and governance frames are taken up but are also subject to resistance, struggles and challenges. Key actors can reconfigure processes, agendas and envisaged identities, reworking their responsibilities and asserting autonomy in the process.

Our first encounters with the 100,000 Genomes Project were at the early stages of our own project when we made contact with some of the project leaders in a nearby region. From the outset we were invited to be part of the development of a consortia bid for a regional genomics medicine centre (GMC), because the practitioners involved were keen to engage us in developing the participatory and evaluative agendas that they viewed as crucial to the success of their bid and the wider initiative. As part of this we attended a meeting with representatives from Genomics England and the NHS where the bid was assessed and discussed, alongside patient representatives, laboratory and service leads and senior managers from relevant hospitals. This encounter, and discussions prior to and following it, were marked by a sense of the need for the practitioners and managers involved to present a suitably ambitious, coherent and compelling case for support, even as they also expressed doubts and concerns in more private settings about the difficulties that this would involve, given other service and resource pressures. In so doing our gatekeepers simultaneously performed the hopeful promissory futures of genomic medicine and service transformation through recruiting practitioners and other allies to participate in the programme delivery, and a more muted set of concerns and ambivalence about the prospects of success for the science and the services involved. The project leaders adopted a kind of strategic uncertainty as part of their negotiation of the demands for practitioner participation, empathising with the doubts and concerns that were also being expressed by colleagues expected to deliver on the initiative.

Our efforts to be part of the project, to follow how it was developed and enacted locally and to share results were, however, constrained by its complex architecture, changing personnel and difficulties of implementation across different cancer clinics, clinical leads and institutions. Jurisdictional disputes around the ownership and purpose of the project were ongoing, as was ambivalence among key actors about their role and its value. We encountered numerous uncertainties about how the project would be delivered. Consent processes were difficult to observe because of ongoing issues with staff training, patients not attending, and clinicians not advising staff about suitable patients. The project was being introduced to a service under strain, where efforts to meet waiting time targets and manage staff absence and well-being came into tension with its delivery. Practitioner participation was patchy, uneven and markedly ambivalent.

The project lead, who was tasked with advocacy for the project, nevertheless framed it as the beginning of a new kind of healthcare based on 'big data' and Artificial Intelligence:

> And the Genomics Project is part of the wider personalised medicine agenda of the NHS, which is a top level objective of the NHS. And very few people really quite get what that means. And in reality what it means is that – it's really a big data project, so it looks like a lab based project but it's actually – actually a project about the, the – about leverage of large datasets. And so the end point of the programme really is that genomics data, er, will be merged with all the other data that can be linked through someone's NHS number into a central data repository.
>
> And from that, tools will be developed that can then apply the, the power of that dataset to the care of individual patients. And that's what really personalised medicine – the personalised medicine agenda is about. And that is an enormous transformation in medical care, um, absolutely huge.

But this was not a view that was widely shared among practitioners concerned about the practicalities of implementation. As another clinician involved in leadership of the project commented:

> in order to know what's relevant to that particular patient at that particular point of time of course you've got to know what their cancer is doing at that particular point in time. So it takes us from a situation where you've … almost got to have a real time readout at any point in time to know what are the particular drivers of … this particular patient's cancer which brings us into personalised medicine … and as exciting as that is, the idea of personalised medicine, the practicalities of that are … really … challenging … financially, organisationally, um, um, diagnostically, therapeutically … in terms of comprehension and understanding (laughs), you know, of, of the clinicians and the population – all of those have … got challenges.

This meant that even as this grander vision of healthcare was being articulated at a range of meetings and events, it was hedged with caveats about the complexities of personalisation, not just in terms of infrastructure, but in terms of the information it brought into clinical practice. As the project lead quoted above continued, the prospects of personalisation and precision were not necessarily straightforward, and could be difficult for practitioners and patients:

> I mean, it's easy if you've got a ninety-five per cent chance of being cured, but if you're saying to somebody, 'Actually, we know from all this data that this is just not going to work,' then that's … something that … people reject. Because if you open the box then you've got the information, if you don't do it in the first place you can just carry on regardless. So that's I think one of the big challenges of this, people see actually personalised medicine as something potentially very, very difficult.

The project leads also spoke of their sense that this project and personalised medicine more generally were 'battling against the biology', revealing much more uncertainty than the rhetoric of precision suggests and that patients might expect, and bringing challenges for practitioners in terms of implementation and interpretation (Metzler 2010).

Practitioners expected to implement the programme in their clinics by supporting patient recruitment also asserted their jurisdiction over healthcare, expressing wariness about top-down initiatives and in the words of one oncologist 'politicians' pet projects', referencing David Cameron's spearheading of the initiative. This oncologist commented: 'Happy to be proved wrong but … I am not a big fan of politicians interfering in healthcare … [with these kinds of initiatives] … we're struggling to pay for other things and I'm not sure it's good value for money.' Others expressed concern about the project being less about evidence-based science than service transformation designed to introduce the automation and centralisation of laboratory services or limit the role of clinicians in interpreting data. This evoked a counter-narrative about the need for clinically embedded analytics, as in the excerpt from an interview with a pathologist below:

> now we … feel strongly that that is in some situations dangerous because a lot of molecular testing is being undertaken by non-clinically … trained geneticists who don't necessarily understand some of the complexities of the material coming in … some centres don't even look at the material that goes through the sequencer so they will, will take sections of pathology material, put it through a box and come

out with an answer and unless you really understand the details of what's gone in, you can't understand the details of what comes out. So we strongly feel that there needs to be a lot more clinical input ... we do have that balance to a degree ... working alongside the genetic clinical scientists to deliver the service so we can provide some clinical oversight ... But other centres will offer blanket clinical interpretations which may not necessarily be appropriate and the problem is oncologists act on those clinical interpretations, not necessarily if they're, if they're up to speed and they're academic and ... they've been to the big meetings recently and they're aware of the evidence and they understand how to interpret the result themselves, but if you're ... a busy general oncologist working in a smaller hospital you're not necessarily up to speed with all the evidence for specific disease types then you make take at face value the clinical interpretations attached to these reports.

Here, concerns about service transformation were reframed not just as about being 'put out of a job', as one pathologist joked, but as a matter of ensuring that current patients benefited from participation. As another pathologist explained with respect to the need to collect fresh tissue for the 100,000 Genomes Project: 'I would put a wager that [fresh tissue] is not that critical for patients in the majority of cases.' Practitioners also expressed ambivalence about the cohort of patients being recruited, as illustrated in this quote from an interview with another pathologist:

not necessarily the right cohort of patients are actually being recruited ... for example, we have recruited a large number of ... GI tumours, but none of those patients will require any sort of treatment and the data that is going to come out from tumour profiling is not going to change how they are managed currently. Now whether it will be managed – whether it will change in the future, we do not know. So ... I've got to be careful about this, so whether it would have been appropriate to actually gather the evidence first and then spend the money building the infrastructure ...

In this excerpt the interviewee intimates that efforts are being made to improve recruitment and meet targets but this is not necessarily involving patients who will directly benefit from the project, as suggested in its design and promotion.

Nurses and one clinical trials assistant (CTA) involved in obtaining participants' consent to the programme had less professional power through which to resist or rework these new agendas. But they were also ambivalent about their role and the prospects of the project. Their ambivalence found particular expression in relation to their concerns about managing project information and encounters with patients, given the complexity of the project. These concerns often took the form of expressions of anxiety or jokes about our presence as observers in the consent meetings, where nurses sought to navigate their sense of being judged or evaluated against an established standard approach to consent where the virtues of the project were largely scripted in advance. Here the nurses framed our presence and that of the project around it as being a new 'script' to learn and implement, positioning themselves as in ongoing need of training and education around genomics to enable the programme to develop.

Nurses also expressed ambivalence about the project with respect to managing patients' expectations around delivery of results. There were significant delays in getting results to patients, and nurses had to field additional phone calls from patients about this, but they had little sense of connection to the 'background' of results being analysed and delivered. At the same time, however, nurses were clearly developing new kinds of expertise and skills in tailoring and navigating the consent process to accommodate patients' needs as part of their ethos of care. We can see some of this play out in an excerpt from an observation of and between consent meetings with patients where a specialist nurse and the GMC specialist nurse discussed their roles and how to support patients:

> The nurses chatted about this patient. The specialist nurse said 'she doesn't sound clued up' and it seemed like the patient was relying on her husband's support [they could hear her husband helping the patient in the background]. Both said it must be particularly difficult for brain cancer patients. They said 'the general gist is that getting sample, helping … and then a bit more of the nitty-gritty. And then ask if they understand.' The specialist nurse said 'you can pick that up'. The GMC specialist nurse said if you feel the patient doesn't comprehend and you are not confident, suggest not to take consent and suggest face-to-face meeting, although they may not be well enough to come in for an extra visit as they will have to drive, park, and wait etc. They added that electronic consent was discussed as a possibility but there was debate around it – not implemented in the end although not clear why. The specialist nurse chipped in by saying

'how do you know people understand?' [when the consent has been done electronically] and went on to suggest that there seem to be 'hiccups' in the project. The GMC specialist nurse said when the study was opened nothing was set up. The specialist nurse asked why? GMC specialist nurse: lots of high level activities went on to set up the Centre. Other Trusts used funding differently to engage nurses but for some there is no job security ... Sounded like lots of people moved on to different work so constantly re-recruit the team and train. They ended up spending lots of her time in rare disease rather than cancer: resources could be better but exciting even though it wasn't up and running when she joined ... The specialist nurse commented: it's like 'giving you a car but not the key, situation' ... The GMC specialist nurse added that she doesn't have a job to go back to [after the end of the 100K project], she is 'not hopeful'.

A lot is going on in this excerpt: the nurses are engaged in training; they are trying to make a complex project work in the absence of guidance and resources, including lack of job security; and, at the same time tailor and make consent meaningful and participation valuable for patients without it becoming too burdensome. This results in a reframing of the project as problematic while maintaining and developing a professional commitment to try to make it work in the interests of patients.

Backstage, practitioners were cautious about the 100,000 Genomes Project, as well as being hopeful about its potential for patients. They wanted genomics to improve treatments for patients, but were sceptical of over-promising and concerned to maintain some of the boundaries between the state and the market that this project was designed to break down. Sometimes these concerns were shared with project leads and the visionary vanguard at events and other meetings. However, we observed that criticism was typically reworked by the project leads as a need for further training or buy-in from staff, or even as a form of professional inertia and protectionism. Difficulties with recruitment became institutional problems and the focus of the national initiative was on successes in terms of numbers of genomes sequenced as a key milestone of progress. In these ways, resistance was itself reworked to form part of the impetus for further transformation of services and institutions.

Practitioner resistance and concerns were also reworked frontstage where patient encounters were concerned, where the focus switched to careful handling of patients' expectations, balancing appeals to patients' altruism and faith in research with management of their hopes and expectations. Practitioners also had to navigate some of the more complex issues around access to data and commercialisation with care, given their qualms about the intricacies and politics of these arrangements. Transformation, however fraught, relied upon practitioners recruiting patients to the project and good care relied upon spending time to reassure and support patients in these and other clinical and research encounters. As we shall now go on to discuss, patients and accompanying relatives were also active participants in these processes, which involved their own resistance and reframing, particularly in relation to informed consent and genomic literacy.

Patient participation

Cancer patients were approached about their involvement in the 100,000 Genomes Project at various points, including before initial surgery or after they had been living with cancer for a number of years (e.g. haematological cancers). They typically received a letter or a phone call inviting them to make an appointment to come along to hear more about the project and to consider participation. These initial encounters with the nurses or CTAs who were trained or in training to conduct the consent appointment lasted up to one hour and covered a range of complex information and deliberation. Patients were often, though not always, accompanied by a family member to these meetings.

A major concern of the project architects was to ensure that patients did not experience participation in this research as too much of a burden and that they understood that receiving potential results of interest to their care, or that of their family members in the future, was contingent on sharing their data and waiving rights to personal financial benefit. This resulted in a detailed consent process which caused concern for practitioners who felt it could be too difficult for patients to manage given their health and other pressures.

In our observations and interviews we found that patients, alongside practitioners, worked to reduce or resist this burden. One way in which this was achieved was by deriving care from the consent meeting. This involved reframing participation from a research experience which might provide better care in the future into an occasion for care in the present. This meant discussions in the meetings could be wide ranging, as patients articulated their experiences and concerns about their cancer, the care they had received, and the prospects of further diagnostic information. The appointments with the consenting nurse or CTA were also a space where patients and family members could discuss immediate, ongoing concerns and worries for the future and to ask questions about their care. None of this was necessarily related to the 100,000 Genomes Project. This included questions about treatment and surgery, as in the following example:

> [After agreeing to take part in the 100,000 Genomes Project] The patient then took out a couple of sheets of paper from her handbag and started to ask the research nurse a series of questions she had prepared. Her questions however were not relevant to the 100,000 Genomes Project but were mostly about her surgery. The research nurse reminded the patient that she can get in touch with a nurse specialist who will be able to answer her questions. … The husband who had been silent then asked a question for the first time, but it was again about the logistics of the patient's surgery: he wanted to know whether he needed to take time off from work. The patient jokingly said to her husband, '[the research nurse] is doing research, not work arrangement' and laughed.

At other times patients sought more practical support, as well as reassurance and advice from the NHS and nurses in particular, as the following example from our observations illustrates:

> The nurse went on to discuss data security and access and how there won't be any financial benefits for patients although it will benefit the NHS. This is normally the point where patients quietly nod or smile/joke … but the patient says, 'some financial help would have been nice; there's no help at all'. And he goes on to talk about how he cannot work but hasn't been offered additional help because his wife is working a few hours a week. The nurse signposted Macmillan nurses to discuss financial issues…
>
> … The nurse then explained the main findings and extra findings e.g. about high cholesterol. The patient says he doesn't worry really but his wife says 'I'm the worrier.' When the nurse explains the genetic carrier testing the patient's wife talked about their decision not to

have children because they were 'too selfish' and wanted to keep enjoying motorbiking …

… the patient asks if people ever come into this meeting but don't want to sign and the nurse says, 'people want to contribute'. His wife agreed about the importance of 'helping future generations', continuing 'breakthroughs happen in science all of the time'. The nurse responded, 'science relies on people like you.' The patient's wife goes on to explain her husband's history of blackouts and a pacemaker being fitted prior to his diagnosis with cancer and wonders if the blackouts were connected to his cancer. The nurse says she cannot answer that question. The patient's wife asks if the project might be able to find out more about this, but the nurse said she was not sure what kind of information was relevant to the project. She added that a copy of the form would be sent to their address and the patient said it will be 'helpful to research but also helpful for my brain' and the nurse added that the overall aim of the project is to 'transform the health service'.

Although these exchanges might be framed as tangential to the core purpose of consent meetings, departing from the framing of the consent protocols and forms, they were key aspects of the meetings which enabled nurses to reciprocate care for patients' involvement, and for patients and family members to generate tangible value from their involvement rather than the remote prospect of personalised results emerging in the future. Being able to articulate positivity and to express concerns, even though the nurses often responded by signposting other kinds of care, was also an opportunity for patients and relatives to perform good patienthood and care giving, bolstering their sense of self-worth in the process. Patients frequently sought the advice of the nurse, or used this unusually lengthy encounter with the nurse to explain their concerns or express gratitude for the care they had received from the NHS. Patients also frequently contextualised the possibility of receiving their results at some point in the future with accounts of their more immediate and pressing concerns about financial issues, pain management and disease progression, for example the question 'Will I be alive by Christmas?'

In so doing, practitioners, patients and family members reconstituted the 'consent to participate' process as a moment of reciprocal care rather than an exercise in deliberation and choice, already generating experiences of care from the encounter rather than awaiting results and future care. As with other encounters with genomic medicine discussed throughout this book, patients situated the 100,000 Genomes Project as but one step on a lengthy and complicated personalised search for care, rather than as a matter of participating in a research project aimed at generating value from their data. This meant that each consent meeting was effectively tailored to different patient experiences, concerns and accounts, as the nurses sought to navigate the encounter as a way of delivering more personal kinds of care and consent. The consent process became an occasion of personalised medicine of a rather more immediate and mundane sort than the high-level, high-tech vision of the programme's leading proponents.

The burden of consent and the specialness of the 100,000 Genomes Project was also resisted by normalising participation as part of 'routine' involvement in other research studies or trials which were integral to being a cancer patient. As one breast cancer patient in the early stages of cancer commented, echoing comments from participants in SMP2 discussed in Chapter 4, 'Why wouldn't I participate? I have no good reason not to.' Another patient, Joe, a former engineer in his sixties who had had surgery and chemotherapy for bowel cancer, commented about donating tissue being an obvious and easy way to help:

> But like I said to (Research Nurse), as long as I don't have to have my leg cut off, or I'm not going to be in pain for weeks and weeks, or I'm not going to be locked up in prison … I [am not] bothered.
>
> **Okay.**
>
> How else are you going to learn [and] advance cancer research … I mean you can't go cutting people up who haven't had cancer just to check, obviously, but … it's the nearest thing you can do with … not live tissue, but with real tissue as opposed to doing it in the classroom.

Other patients, especially those who had recently had surgery or those who were about to have it, told us that getting rid of the tumour – 'why would I want it?' – by donating it to the project was an easy decision, perhaps as part of a wider effort to show their willingness to participate.

Reframing participation as obvious and routine, as opposed to special and burdensome, allowed patients and their relatives to maintain self-worth in the face of cancer, asserting their agency and dignity as well as their care and concern for future patients. But in other respects we saw that participation was not routine – not only was the meeting quite time consuming, it also involved logistics such as transport and parking, enrolling relatives into the process. Patients and their relatives nevertheless made this workable by coordinating their involvement alongside other appointments at the hospital. This articulation work was key to the successful recruitment of patients to the project. For instance, one elderly patient, Brigit, who was frail and forgetful due to her recent major brain surgery, told us that if consenting to the 100,000 Genomes Project or speaking with us had required 'special trips' to the hospital, she would not have participated as she relied on her sons and a daughter-in-law to take turns to drive her to hospital. On the day of the consent meeting, her daughter-in-law accompanied Brigit, and when we interviewed her on a different day one of her sons had taken the day off to accompany her for a clinic appointment. In the interview they told us they were happy to help 'as long as things like this interview could fit in with when we're here'. Brigit also explained her desire to participate in the consent meeting to her son:

> And I just said, 'Well, I – as I told you, I was gonna do this,' and I just says to him, 'Don't forget … it's something that I want to do,' I said, 'But I'm not at a position where I can go like talking to anybody or go here or [there or] anything like that,' I says, 'But on paper I can do it.' So that's … was basically it, you know…

This reworking of participation as routine and unremarkable was also associated with ideas of their data already being available elsewhere and research of this sort as a social good which might also benefit the patient, and future patients, including family members.

Arranging an interview with one patient, Giles, was difficult because he was adapting to living with some complications after his surgery while undergoing a phased return to his work as a data scientist. However, Giles was particularly keen to participate, telling us he would have felt he was being 'hypocritical' if he refused. He told us that he already knew about the project and was confident it was beneficial:

> I'd heard, I'd heard of it on a … level when I worked for the [name of company where the patient works], but I didn't know any details

of it. So I knew, I knew such a thing existed and they were gathering genetics on people with cancer for future study.

So when [you were] formally approached by health professionals, did you, did you find more about the 100,000 Genomes Project then?

They gave me … plenty of information but I didn't read a lot of it … I knew enough to know that it was a beneficial study based on genetics of cancer. And I didn't see any reason not to take part in such a thing and I didn't feel the need to learn more details about what I was helping with because I was happy to help.

He also saw data sharing as an unproblematic: 'I don't believe that storing data on people is going to cause me a disaster … I mean I didn't pay that much attention to the opt-out process because I wasn't particularly worried about it, or the data protection issues…' Giles went on to 'call out' people who worry about this because of the acceptance of surveillance in everyday life, and even its inevitability: 'The ones selling [data] to people are not the NHS – it's Facebook and Google … And if the government wants to spy on me they will regardless of whether or not I've signed a consent form!' Another older breast cancer patient, Ally, introduced in Chapter 2, explained that she had chosen to participate in the hope that genomic information that might help her extended family would be uncovered:

it outweighs the thought of, oh somebody's got my details, for goodness sake, everybody has got people's details nowadays … your mobile phone, if you've got your location on that, big brother is watching you! … at the end of the day, if you've done nothing wrong, what is there to worry about?

Patients were much more concerned with the practicalities of participation such as whether it might involve more hospital visits, than about data security. Through these kinds of narratives participants were not necessarily expressing strong commitment to the project, including trust in its data security arrangements, but a sense that participation was not likely to be problematic, especially given that data is already being shared in ways we inevitably have little control over, by governments and corporations (Zuboff 2019). By actively not worrying about these kinds of things they once again asserted their self-worth as rational and sensible citizens willing to help others. The only exception to this concerned the possibility that insurance companies might access data, which can be a source of concern for participants, as has been established through a range of survey and consultation exercises.[10] The nurses therefore sought to incorporate information about this – for example, the moratorium in place – in the consent procedures. We noticed that as similar questions were asked at each meeting they presented this information upfront even before the related questions were raised by participants.

We also found that where concerns did arise, these were often softened afterwards. For example, Lillian, introduced in Chapter 2, explained how she and her husband were initially wary of private, for-profit companies accessing her genomic data when this came up in the consent meeting:

> it was a bit of a knee jerk reaction … a lot of commercial organisations kind of jump on the bandwagon … to get your information … to prey on people … and once it's gone outside this kind of ethical boundary … But then of course, I know that most medical research is done by this kind of company, when I thought about it, I thought, well how stupid. Private companies, they're the ones that have got the finances … to put into medical research.

Here, being a good participant meant reflecting back on excess reactions and accepting the role of market forces and privatisation in genomic research.

Patients and relatives engaged with the information provided, including before and during the consent meeting, in a range of ways, sometimes asking a lot of questions or commenting on their own expertise in a related field to reinforce their understanding, and at other times disengaging or resisting a lot of information. For example: 'The patient says she does research in an allied health field so she understands ethics and consent. She added that personalised medicine has been practised in her field for a long time and for her "genomics" is too "medical" a term to describe this.' Here, the patient establishes that she has sufficient expertise to make informed decisions.

Resisting information was another strategy we observed, when participants might wave away the consent form or interrupt the nurse to say they were happy to sign without her going through her scripted explanation. Participants also sometimes commented about there being too much information – 'like an examination!' – but laughed this off or didn't read all the material because it would 'take all day', and went ahead and consented. When asked about the information previously provided, a colorectal patient in his late forties, Stevie, commented: 'I read it. Don't ask me about it 'cause I can't remember.' Nevertheless, Stevie expressed his excitement and interest in the 100,000 Genomes Project, telling us he was 'fascinated' and looking forward to seeing the results. This is also illustrated in the following extract from one of our observations of a consent meeting:

> The nurse asks how they were informed about the project and they say it was a letter through the post. The patient's wife then took the consent form out of the envelope. The patient says, 'I haven't read it', with a big smile, and the nurse answers, 'don't worry, we'll be talking it through'. The patient says he is not an expert and not a medic so 'do whatever you want to do'. He says he knows how to mend bikes but not mend brains. When the nurse asks if his tumour has been removed they both say 'biopsy' and the patient went on to say 'they wanted to drill but realised my brain wasn't that big' and we all laughed.

In these kinds of interactions humour was deployed as a mechanism through which participants could mediate their lack of knowledge and understanding while also building rapport with clinical professionals and bolstering their identity as a competent participant.

Participants also complied with, but subtly reworked, the educational aspect of the consent process by adopting the position of critical observer or media consumer when viewing the accompanying video used as part of the consent process, often nodding appreciatively or commenting on its quality, for example 'very well put together'. In another consultation, we observed the following:

> The 4-minute video clip played, and the couple watched it with concentration. Both smiled especially at the 'Giant Super Secure Database' section [explaining the security of the 100,000 Genomes database]. Once the clip ended both smiled and the patient's husband said 'Excellent! Sorry, that [video] answered my questions.'

Together these kinds of encounters and discourses reframed the consent process as an occasion for care and the performance of gratitude, competency and good patienthood.

Participation was also sometimes rationalised as a way of keeping practitioners on side to keep care foregrounded even when it was lacking, something that takes more work than giving consent. For example, one breast cancer patient, Nicky, a healthcare practitioner and teacher who had lived with cancer for over a decade, told us how she was not concerned when her consent meeting was very short with little time for reflection or discussion (because the nurse was not experienced in the consent process for cancer patients):

> to me it was just signing the forms, honestly ... it's funny, I think because I've had so many different experiences and positive and negative ... you don't get angry any more about if – if you're not treated in the best way that you could do. You know, I used to get really angry at the start if I got bad care or someone wasn't treating me, you know, right and, you know, and ... to be honest, I just let it go now because, you know, people have bad days. People struggle, you know. There's lots of stuff going off and really if I kicked up a fuss and got arsy, it makes ... no joy for anybody, least of all me really ... you've gotta work with these people and you might meet them again in the future, so that plays on your mind as well. Might it affect my future care, future, you know, how that person responds and is with me? Um, it shouldn't do that, but ... you do think about that.

This extract shows that patients situated their consent to this project in relation to a much lengthier ongoing experience with cancer and care. For some, participation in this project faded into the background of ongoing efforts to stay well, but in this case, it could also be a form of investment in future care and good relations with care staff.

These ways of reducing the burden of consenting to participate and deriving care in the present or future complement the efforts of those involved in the governance of the project to simplify and shorten the consent process as a way of ensuring higher levels of participation in the project. But they also trouble the model of consent in the project governance, where emphasis is placed upon patients engaging with the project on its own terms and being fully cognisant of the waiver of their rights to financial benefits, and the limited opportunities for results which will direct their care. Instead they involve patients by strategically ignoring or discounting the ways in which data and profit flow in the project, and importantly and empathetically searching for care within this encounter.

Through these practices, patients subtly reworked the governing frames of the 100,000 Genomes Project by turning the consent meeting into an occasion to display a good enough level of expertise about genomics and cancer. This was an exercise in preserving dignity and competency as a person, not just a cancer patient. We see this kind of work as part of patients constituting themselves as worthy-of-a-future, where care would continue to be offered and received on a reciprocal basis. Together these practices reclaimed dignity in a kind of ordinary personhood as distinct from a more educated patienthood which the 100,000 Genomes Project seeks to cultivate. At the same time, however, the overarching knowledge-control regime is enacted rather than undermined via these reworked forms of participation, as data is collected and participation is valued as a personal and social good.

Conclusion

The next stage in the mainstreaming of genomic medicine in the NHS, the development of the Genomics Medicine Service in England, aims to put the service in 'pole position' to make use of the technology, according to Dame Sue Hills, Chief Scientific Officer for England. Genomics once again became a key reference point in politicians' vision for the service in 2018, as in this quote from Matt Hancock, the newly appointed Health and Social Care Minister: 'The power of genomics plus AI to use the NHS's data to save lives is literally greater than anywhere else on the planet.' Initially, however, WGS will only be available for some rare diseases and 'hard to treat cancers', with an aspiration to sequence one million genomes by the NHS and UK Biobank within a year, and up to five million by the Genomics Medicine Service within five years. Illumina and other companies involved in organising and interpreting genomic data are key to turning what Hills described as the 'cottage industry' of genomic laboratories into 'factories [with] higher quality, faster throughput and turn-round, and cheaper prices', in her evidence to the House of Commons Science and Technology Committee inquiry into genomics in the NHS. But we remain unclear about how these 'factories' will deliver the benefits of expensive targeted therapies to a cash-strapped NHS once it has delivered its genomic data to the commercial market.

Genomic sequencing initiatives at a national scale are a major part of the bioeconomy and the personalisation of healthcare for common diseases such as cancer. For countries such as the UK, being a key part of these developments is crucial to economic growth and prosperity. To cultivate these values, a genomic vanguard has sought to leverage one of the UK's true great assets, the NHS, transforming the service to embed genomic data collection and analysis across its cancer clinics and beyond. Patient participation on a large scale is vital to success, but the burdens and benefits of participation must be carefully circumscribed as part of the new era of reflexive governance, as patients' data is being put to work in the national interest. Scientists, clinicians and social researchers are recruited into this task to develop appropriate methods of govern-ance and understand how patients participate in order to improve levels of participation, including via enhanced levels of genomic literacy.

Patients and their families participate in these initiatives willingly, but the terms of their participation are reworked in the process as the value they realise consolidates around care in the moment and giving back to carers and future patients. Patients resist the burden of consent by asserting a good enough level of knowledge or normalising participation as a routine part of hospital visits and engagement with care givers. Their engagement with the economic value that their participation might generate is, however, curtailed, in a complex consent process which evokes trust in practitioners and providers to use their data for the common good. Facing a difficult diagnosis, or recovering from major surgery, patients are vulnerable, sometimes confused and emotional about their experiences and participation, and keen to make a good impression on the nurses who take them through the consent process. Staff also find ways of resisting and reworking the governing frames of the project, including consent and recruitment processes, prioritising care during consent meetings and querying efforts to improve recruitment and reorganise services backstage of clinical and policy encounters. Their resistance can, however, give further impetus to the genomic vanguard's efforts to intensify transformation, locating responsibility for change with institutions already experiencing a range of financial and service pressures.

Notes

1 https://assets.publishing.service.gov.UK/government/uploads/system/ uploads/attachment_data/file/213705/dh_132382.pdf (accessed 20 June 2020).

2 www.mckinsey.com/business-functions/digital-mckinsey/our-insights/ disruptive-technologies (accessed 20 June 2020).

3 The Institute of Fiscal Studies reports that 'The period between 2009–10 and 2014–15 saw historically slow increases in UK public spending on health, averaging 1.1% per year. This was the lowest five-year growth rate since a consistent time series of health spending began in 1955–56. However, due to cuts in other services, health spending continued to increase as a share of public service spending.' www.ifs.org.UK/ publications/8879 (accessed 20 June 2020).

4 Genomics England press release, 'UK to become world number one in DNA testing with plan to revolutionise fight against cancer and rare disease', 1 August 2014.

5 https://youtu.be/UL-K1_Z0vmc (accessed 20 June 2020).

6 https://assets.publishing.service.gov.UK/government/uploads/system/ uploads/attachment_data/file/210830/ethics_advice_letter_to_CMO.pdf (accessed 20 June 2020).

7 www.genomicsengland.co.UK/wp-content/uploads/2018/10/genomics_ public_dialogue_ipsos_mori_literature_review.pdf (accessed 20 June 2020).

8 www.genomicsengland.co.UK/public-dialogue-report-published/ (accessed 20 June 2020).

9 'As the NHS celebrates 70 years Genomics England sequences its 70,000th genome', 4 July 2018, https://www.genomicsengland.co.uk/ as-the-nhs-celebrates-70-years-genomics-england-sequences-its-70000th-genome/ (accessed 20 June 2020).

10 www.genomicsengland.co.UK/wp-content/uploads/2018/10/genomics_ public_dialogue_ipsos_mori_literature_review.pdf (accessed 20 June 2020).

6

Going private: digital culture and personalised medicine

Tensions around the value generated by the complicated nexus of private, public and industry arrangements of large-scale genomic sequencing initiatives can also be found in the wider political economy of targeted therapies. Personalised cancer drugs promise cures and economic growth. But their expense presents a problem for healthcare providers and patients alike. Recent reports suggest that in one of the largest markets, the USA, spending on cancer drugs in the genomic era has increased dramatically – rising from $26 billion in 2012 to more than $45 billion in 2016, with targeted therapies accounting for 60 per cent of this increase (Bekelman and Joffe 2018). Others report that prices for targeted cancer therapies can be as much as $350,000 per patient per year (Tiriveedhi 2018: 36, quoting Gavan et al. 2018: 1). In insurance-based healthcare systems such as that in the USA, where not everyone is covered for these kinds of treatments, this is plunging families into debt. Authors have written about the 'financial toxicity' that accompanies the chemical toxicity of cancer drugs, with the American Centers for Disease Control and Prevention reporting that one in three US citizens experience financial difficulties due to medical care, with the greatest burden falling on cancer patients who face a range of so-called 'out of pocket expenses' for cancer; for example, it has been reported that 13 per cent of non-elderly patients spend over 20 per cent of their income on out-of-pocket expenses (Zafar 2015: 370).

For many cancer patients and their families, this is a price worth paying. Targeted drugs are also prized by the genomic vanguard (Hilgartner 2017) that we discussed in the previous chapter, who argue that personalisation will grow the economy and save the health service money as drugs are targeted more effectively. But even in established and well-regarded public healthcare systems such as the NHS, it is difficult to meet these ballooning costs. 'Buying in' to this promissory future involves a costly 'embrace' of biomedicine. As Good notes,

> While the world's dominant economies invest private and public monies in the production of biotechnology and aggressively seek to integrate these advances into clinical practice – thereby reaping financial as well as scientific returns on [often tax-funded] capital investments – all societies are confronted with difficult questions about rationing biomedical interventions assumed central to competent clinical medicine. (2001: 407)

In the UK this is made more complex by different decision-making arrangements across England, Wales and Scotland. NICE, the body responsible for deciding what treatments will be made available to patients in England, operates a Cancer Drugs Fund, a managed access scheme which tries to ensure that patients get early access to promising treatments and to encourage 'responsible pricing' by pharmaceutical companies to ensure value for money for the public purse.[1] The Scottish Medicines Consortium advises NHS Scotland on the clinical merits and cost-effectiveness of new medicines. In many ways this arrangement reflects public opinion on the need to try to manage cancer drug costs in the same way as treatments for other conditions.[2] However, bodies making funding decisions are also heavily criticised by cancer patients and their supporters when they are faced with a decision not to fund hoped-for treatments. There are numerous stories in the media of patients and families affected by these kinds of decisions criticising 'NHS bureaucrats' and the 'postcode lottery'. As we write, one such story has hit the headlines. This is the case of an NHS worker with advanced cervical cancer who lives in Wales. She has been denied access to Avastin, a targeted therapy, by the All-Wales Medicines Strategy Group, but if she lived in England she would be able to access the drug via the Cancer Drugs Fund.[3]

Aside from these difficulties about the fairness and consistency of decision making across the UK, funding decisions are also beset by a range of problems regarding how to evaluate and establish what counts as an effective treatment. There is no shortage of economic formulae designed to work out what should be funded based on cost and clinical effectiveness. But this is not an area where formulae are enough to satisfy the complex needs of patients, advocates and practitioners. So disputes abound about how to calculate benefit and what kinds of evidence count in this process. Of course, such disagreements are common across decision making around tests and treatments for an array of different diseases, not just cancer. There is also a long history of drugs being expensive and experimental in cancer care. But personalised cancer medicines make this situation even more complicated and difficult for three main reasons. First, the idea of personalisation brings with it a sense of individual patients' entitlement to new and experimental treatments; not being treated as one of the 'herd' but as special and deserving of the opportunity to take the risk. This increases patient pressure on the decision-making body. Second, these therapies are, by their very nature, experimental, and as such there is limited evidence of effectiveness. The impetus to be permissive rather than restrictive is part of a wider experimental ethos perpetuated through major charitable institutions that fund cancer research – institutions that are embedded in the fabrics of our lives via a plethora of fundraising initiatives and charitable giving. This further increases pressure on decision makers. Third, and perhaps most importantly, personalised medicines are most effective for particular subgroups of patients, depending on their genomic profile, and yet evidence of this benefit can be difficult to generate. The way in which the effectiveness of cancer therapies is evaluated tends to rely on a lot of evidence of benefit across larger or mixed groups of patients. Gathering the right kind of evidence to satisfy the requirements of decision-making bodies is difficult because it means having to work out, in advance, what kinds of patients might benefit more than others and to put trials and studies into place to ensure that the drugs can be given consistently and safely, and monitored properly, to amass sufficient evidence. Patient pathways and trial arrangements are complex and cancers can progress quickly, making these kinds of studies difficult to conduct. Cancer is a complex and evolving disease, so the era of personalised medicine is not just about finding a one-off 'wonder drug' that makes all the difference. Instead, cancer therapies are offered in combination, and these combinations shift over time as the cancer evolves. This makes the benefits of one particular drug even more difficult to establish, putting researchers and funding decision makers in a kind of Catch-22 situation: evidence of benefit is required but is difficult to establish because treatments are not yet permitted.

Behind the headlines about the revolutionary potential of personalised cancer medicines to cure cancer, there are complex and difficult stories of the benefits, and drawbacks, of targeted therapies. These therapies can give patients a few extra precious months or years of life, but is that enough to justify their high cost to the NHS? As Bekelman and Joffe recently discussed in the *Journal of the American Medical Association*, cancer drugs rarely show substantial improvements in life expectancy. They give the example of neratinib, a drug for patients with early-stage breast cancer, which has been shown to improve 'invasive disease-free survival' by 2 per cent. The monthly cost of this drug is $10,500 (Bekelman and Joffe 2018: 2167). For experts and citizens this can be too high a price to pay for marginal gain, but other patients and relatives contest these kinds of calculations, pointing to other evidence they have gathered from their own experiences and those of fellow cancer patients, which shows that they are living longer and better lives because of these kinds of drugs. From the 'exceptional responders' we sometimes see in the media, to their own experiences and discussions with patients and practitioners online and in person, cancer patients and their advocates can draw on this more diffuse, informal evidence to build a sense that the bureaucratic calculus of 'benefit' is unimaginative, perhaps even callous.

Another important feature of this prevailing sense of ambivalence, disappointment and frustration around the cost and availability of personalised cancer medicines is criticism of the predatory pricing and high profits of pharmaceutical companies. Concerns about the spiralling costs of precision medicine have been expressed in a range of quarters. In the journal *Nature Biotechnology*, Schellekens et al. criticise what they see as an 'outmoded' process of drug regulation, but they also state that 'the main contributor to soaring costs is innovation in a market that is driven by what is offered, rather than by medical need' (Schellekens et al. 2017: 507). Cancer charities also become involved in lobbying around pricing strategy. For example, the CRUK website ran a story about pricing, quoting Professor Richard Sullivan, director of the Institute of Cancer Policy at King's College London: 'Pricing is out of hand … The cost basis of what's happening to medicines is very elastic – the prices just keep going up. It's not about value but what the market can bear.'[4]

Although it is widely acknowledged that the cost to companies of developing targeted therapies is high, concerns have been raised among US practitioners that big pharma is not actually spending as much of its profits on research and development as is sometimes claimed, for example by spending on marketing rather than research.[5] NICE and other government bodies, as well as economists and other academics involved in the review and evaluation of drug pricing, have had to be cautious about how they manage this disgruntlement, given how embedded these companies are in government plans for the life sciences economy as a means of boosting UK wealth. However, resistance to the high costs of precision medicine does emerge in negotiations around drug approvals, as part of a wider set of lobbying around access and pricing by patients and advocates. For example, in the face of considerable pressure from cancer charities and patient advocates, NICE negotiated over a number of years with Roche, the manufacturer of a cancer drug called Kadcyla for advanced breast cancer, before granting approval; this reportedly involved an undisclosed discount from the £90,000 ($115,000) per patient cost.[6]

In this chapter we explore what it means to be a cancer patient or advocate caught up in these systems of pricing, evaluation and access. How do patients and their supporters navigate access to targeted drugs that might be inaccessible via the NHS? What kinds of alliances and work does this involve? How does it feel to be told you can only access a treatment on which you have pinned your hopes by paying, or to find that you cannot benefit from this treatment despite having raised significant amounts of money from family and friends to do just that?

Cancer patients, many of whom are younger patients with a late diagnosis, together with their advocates, doctors and campaigners are increasingly seeking access to personalised cancer medicine via a range of routes. As we have already discussed, these include companies' compassionate use schemes and research trials. But it can also involve self- and crowdfunding, alongside appeals against Clinical Commissioning Group decisions and more public challenges to company pricing structures. These activities have blossomed online in the genomic era, among new and established groups of cancer patients and supporters, some of whom have formed alliances around types or stages of cancers, treatments and/or locale in their efforts to improve access to targeted chemotherapies.

Accessing and advocating for experimental therapies involves new biosocial arrangements. These bring patients and advocates together to campaign collectively and build a shared identity around cancer subtypes where experimental drugs offer hope but are not routinely available as part of NHS care. Survivorship as craft (Frank 2003) involves telling one's story and cultivating communities and responsibilities for fellow survivors. These activities also involve new kinds of expertise in advocacy and fundraising, extending entrepreneurial patienthood into the digital world of crowdfunding and profile raising. Digital media platforms are increasingly important means by which patients are active and engaged in these collective and individual battles (Lupton 2014; see also Vicari and Cappai 2016). These form part of what Zuboff (2019) has called 'surveillance capitalism', where profit is derived from tracking, predicting and conditioning user behaviours, often without their knowledge. Cancer patients are actively involved in these platforms as they seek and offer support and advocacy around living with cancer, participating in research and accessing information, tests, treatments and care (Ziebland and Wyke 2012; Ross et al. 2019). Western-centric tropes of survivorship, prioritising enablement, self-responsibility and cheerfulness are common, notably in breast cancer forums (Orgad 2005). As Petersen et al. (2019) argue, there is also growing emphasis in patient campaigning online, where patients work with science and business on profile raising and fundraising. These activities are amplified and monetised by traditional and digital media which 'align with a consumer-driven model of digital patient activism' (Petersen et al. 2019: 489). Facebook and other social media platforms such as Instagram are where patients become involved in what Gerlitz and Helmond have called the 'like economy', where 'like buttons enable multiple data flows between various actors, contributing to a simultaneous de- and re-centralisation of the web' (Gerlitz and Helmond 2013: 1248).

We explore these activities by analysing 15 patients' social media and press coverage and eight interviews with a range of mainly non-NHS patients and their advocates, including patients seeking or self-funding targeted cancer treatments that have been refused or not provided as part of standard NHS care. The interviews were carried out between September 2018 and March 2019. They included patients and their supporters crowdfunding for these treatments using online platforms, campaigners advocating for access and a small number of patients who had gone public about their experiences of self-funding treatments. We also included patients who have accessed private medicine via their medical insurance schemes, typically provided as part of their employment benefits, some of whom avoid speaking about this in public.

These new arrangements transcend categories such as industry-backed 'patient groups' and 'adversarial consumerism' (Williams et al. 2011) and rework theories of biosociality which foreground active partnerships between rare-disease communities and healthcare providers. Instead, following Frank (2003) we argue that these practices of private patienthood are creating and breaking down solidarities in novel and important ways. We highlight digital platforms as a key aspect of these processes, as the sites through which patients and their advocates join each other alongside charities, pharmaceutical companies, universities and healthcare institutions in constituting these new kinds of patienthood. But rather than being wholly benign, these platforms are part of the process of value creation, and are themselves extracting yet more value from patient behaviour now rendered digital. Crucially, we consider how these processes work via appeals to and accounts of the sorts of futures these patients and supporters craft for themselves and others as part of these new social and economic formations, as they try to live well in prognosis.

Private healthcare as right and wrong: personal futures and the future of the NHS

Private cancer medicine in the UK is a significant business. As pressure on NHS funding increases and the regulatory hurdles outlined above multiply, NHS cancer patients are increasingly faced with restrictions on the kinds of drugs they might seek as part of their care. For many NHS patients, this is not an issue – they accept the treatments on offer or join trials to access more experimental therapies. For a growing group of patients, however, private medicine is their main option.

Going private is not necessarily to the exclusion of NHS care, but often patched together with NHS services, typically when patients are able to access private medicine through a workplace insurance scheme. As this patient advocate for ovarian cancer, Sara, explains, this does not necessarily involve speedier access to tests, results and treatment:

> **How did you go about getting a genetic test?**
>
> So I … think I raised it with my oncologist and … requested that I was referred for it. And he … was keen to make that referral. But I was seeing my oncologist privately … [I] think genetic testing, that was through the NHS … I think there was probably some delay because perhaps … I wasn't having my treatment at the time on the NHS and then there were some complications with them having an old address on file … So it probably took about 12 months … from me initiating the conversation to actually having the test, which was a little bit frustrating. But … I got there in the end and I know there's plenty of people who want genetic testing and struggle … to get it.

On the other hand, private medicine did bring Sara privileged access to certain therapies, such as Avastin, a biological therapy which has shown some success for particular groups of cancer patients such as those with a BRAF mutation:

> because I was private, I was, I was having my surgery and my treatment privately, I was automatically eligible for Avastin.
>
> **Did you go private because it was covered by your work?**
>
> Yeah, it was … I initially went to an out of hours doctor based at a local NHS hospital and I was admitted there and had a lot of my initial tests and diagnosis there. And then my follow-up appointment was with the surgeon of that hospital, and when he said the next step is to have a hysterectomy, he said, 'I can do it in three weeks on the NHS or I can do it in a week privately.' And I had the benefit of private cover – so it'd be the same individual doing it, so it wasn't as if I was getting any more – anybody any more skilled or less skilled, but at the time my reaction to it was I just want whatever is in there out of me as soon as, and it felt – because at the time one of the symptoms, I was quite bloated and it seemed to be getting – my stomach seemed to be getting bigger with like fluid, it was almost I just needed whatever it was out.

... But one of the things – so whilst the follow-up treatment I've had privately, one thing that they haven't got is the sort of support services that go around it, so I have been able to access the NHS for a psychologist. I went for reflexology whilst I was having treatment, somebody to talk about benefit, some – my Macmillan nurse was based at the hospital, so I have sort of taken bits from private and public sector, so I've been lucky to do that.

So going back to the question about Avastin, I think because I ... had that cover, there wasn't any question about it ... I don't know whether I would have been eligible had I been NHS ... I don't think it's necessarily routinely available to everybody, there's certain criteria, it might differ depending where geographically you live. So I do feel fortunate that I had the cover and was able to get that without question.

One particular group of patients who are seeking access to drugs not currently available on the NHS are advanced bowel cancer patients who are on their third or fourth line of treatment and would also like to access Avastin. This is not currently funded by the NHS because NICE has not approved access to the treatment due to what is considered insufficient evidence of benefit. But as with the case of the ovarian cancer patient above, some bowel cancer patients have been prescribed the drug privately, pointing to its availability in other countries and a small but growing evidence base that supports its use. These patients have the support of some of the larger charities for this cancer, although there is not a wide-spread campaign as we saw with other high-profile challenges to NICE decisions about targeted treatments, such as from the breast cancer patient community.

Some patients, such as Lydia, access this drug through private medicine because they have insurance, often as part of their workplace benefits. Lydia, a young woman in her thirties diagnosed with advanced bowel cancer, did not experience many of the difficulties with getting a quick diagnosis and access to expensive treatments that she knows other people in her situation face, despite the relative rarity of her case. Lydia, like Sara, told us she was fortunate to have private healthcare insurance and has had access to the best surgeons, oncologists and treatments. She was able to choose to take Avastin alongside other chemotherapy drugs because the alternative treatment protocol might have harmed her ability to continue with her sporting pursuits. This personalised care was more important to Lydia than the 'numbers on the page' about her particular cancer subtype. Lydia found the molecular information difficult to process and told us she avoided trying to find out too much about it as it was overwhelming. She felt very fortunate to be receiving private care, but it also brought a sense of guilt that she had to manage, partly by participating in other research and awareness-raising activities around prevention. Lydia felt that it was wrong that she should be able to benefit from excellent care whereas others could not because some unnamed persons were 'acting like God' to restrict treatments for some NHS patients. Her guilt also meant she kept what she felt was her privileged position as a private cancer patient secret and did not disclose this to other patients in her online community.

Other patients with private healthcare insurance switched to and from NHS and private medicine depending on their needs. This movement between public and private provision is a feature of the current system, as there is choice embedded in NHS service delivery alongside rationing. Alongside major private hospitals, some NHS hospitals might run private patient units (PPUs), including for cancer. These PPUs have an ambiguous position in the NHS, offering a quicker scan or a treatment not available on the NHS but also, as Guy has pointed out, sometimes being advertised as offering the opportunity to patients to help the NHS by reducing the strain on the service (Guy 2019). We interviewed another patient, Rachel, who, like Sara, had switched back and forth between NHS care and private care and was now receiving targeted therapies funded by her insurer which would not otherwise be available on the NHS. Rachel's story illustrates the complexity of these transitions and the feelings these evoke, captured in this lengthy extract:

> at the time it was … I was a bit like a deer in the headlights, as you can imagine … I didn't know anything about cancer. I mean none of my family had had cancer … I was so completely inexperienced with any of it, but I was doing quite a lot of reading … on my condition and the different treatments available to me, and that's when things started to, for me, become a little bit clear that actually … there might be something better for me out there. But actually, I'm not on it because I'm under the NHS.
>
> … I did actually mention it to doctor but … to be honest with you … she'd pretty much written me off … that's a common factor

for a lot of people that find themselves at stage four ... with all the NHS pressures, that actually it's 'well you're terminal anyway ... we're doing our best, it is what it is' ... that didn't really sit that well with me, as you can imagine (laughs softly) so, I transferred my care [to another hospital].

But I, again I transferred as an NHS patient ... and I sat down with my oncologist on the ... first day and said to him, 'Look, am I, am I actually on the best treatment here, or could I be on something better?' And he said, 'No, you're on the best treatment.' And I said, 'Well look, I've, I've read about this thing called Avastin, this drug called Avastin. Is it not worth [trying], because of my BRAF mutation?' ... and he said to me, 'Well, it's very expensive ... so don't worry about it too much ... it's not really that big a deal.' And I said to him, 'Well look, I'm ... I'm potentially a private patient, I've just not really looked into that too much. I don't really know much about the ... private system, and I've got it through work.' And he said, 'Well look, go and speak to – who are you with?' and I said, [name of insurer] and he said, 'Well look, speak to them and see, see if you've got, see if you're covered, and if you are, let me know.' And I did. And they said to me, 'Yes, yeah, we would, we would absolutely fund Avastin,' and I was like, 'Okay, fine.'

Then, I emailed my oncologist to say, 'They've said they will fund me. I'm fully covered,' and he ... phoned back within, between ten minutes and half an hour, and ... the whole conversation completely changed. It was very much, 'This is incredible. Absolutely, we need to get you on Avastin. Avastin really should be available on the NHS anyway, but it isn't because, ... NICE haven't approved it. But it is a standard of care across major, other major countries in the world.'

And I think ... that for me, I found quite shocking and ... quite unfair really because it's not like, I think it's very separate to people being on clinical trials and new drugs coming along ... But a drug that's actually approved across all the other major countries, you know, with the, with the best performing healthcare systems in the world, you know, and it's not approved here. And actually the, the criteria and the justification from NICE I don't think particularly stacks up. Um, and that's, again that's something that, that my oncolog[ist] said to me, he said, you know, 'The, the problem is that the overall data isn't that great, but actually it's good for specific types of colon cancer. And actually, yours is one of them, so we should put you on that,' ... which was, which was great. ... I've been on that ever since.

But I've got lots and lots of friends now who are BRAF mutated and, actually quite scarily, what, what I'm tending to find is that the majority of BRAF patients are, they, they tend to be a lot younger. They tend to be the younger lot and actually these are the ones that can withstand much greater, much stronger treatment and give themselves a much better opportunity and best chance in life to at least have, you know, I don't know, three or four years rather than the one or two that they're being handed.

Um, so the frustration for me is that the, the guideline ... haven't been approved in the correct way, I don't think ... the whole thing has been looked at in, in the most appropriate way ... So I'm, I'm very fortunate, but I've got lots of friends now who are – I've got one chap in particular and he's literally raising money for each session and it's costing him about £1,800 every two weeks. So that's quite frustrating.

Rachel found the guilt and anger at this injustice difficult to manage alone, and this spurred her to write a blog and set up a closed group on Facebook to share her experiences and support other patients to identify the best treatment options depending on their molecular subtype. She spoke about the need for patients to realise that their NHS doctors were operating with 'one hand tied behind their backs!' as part of her efforts to encourage patients to be more active and challenging so that they got the best care. This work sat outside of the more positive, moderated zones of the main charity in this area and included discussion about a range of alternative treatments alongside conventional medicine and targeted treatments. Rachel also spoke about her belief in the NHS and her distress that it was not being given sufficient funds to provide these more expensive treatments. Through these accounts Rachel balanced her identity as a private patient against her sense of biosociality with other similar patients as well as her citizenship and support for public services such as the NHS.

Other patients we interviewed were either already self-funding or planning to pay for treatments themselves. The scale of this market is difficult to quantify, but a recent report estimated that 'the market in self paying patients was heading for "double digit growth" over the next few years and that this was fuelled by longer NHS waiting lists, curbs on access to NHS treatments, and rising private medical insurance premiums'.[7] Some of these patients were able to afford to self-fund without doing things such as remortgaging their homes. One such patient was Phil, another advanced bowel cancer patient, who was self-funding Avastin. Phil was part of an online community of cancer patients and supported the work of one of the main charities for bowel cancer. Like Rachel, he had become something of a public patient through a blog and presence on social media, and his posts included discussion about self-funding the drug which referenced his sense of being fortunate that he was able to find this money. Phil also engaged with more political discussions around NHS resources and funding, including retweeting posts by other advocates about the need to make his treatment more widely available on the NHS. But Phil's decision to self-fund Avastin was careful and contingent, and he was aware of the uncertainties involved:

> I suppose it's a difficult one, isn't it? I mean … it's hard to … know. I suppose from my perspective, I kind of thought, look, you know, I'm in a situation where I've got advanced bowel cancer … I can afford to do it, fortunately, so I thought, well, you know, although it's expensive, I'm gonna, you know, give it a whirl. You know, I don't want to … die wondering whether … it would've made a difference or not. And I think one of the problems … with Avastin is it's difficult to measure what the effectiveness of the drug is. … I'm taking it alongside chemotherapy and … if the overall treatment's effective, it's, it's not really possible to … measure whether the effectiveness is through the chemo or through the Avastin … But, you know, I thought … I'm gonna give it a go for this cycle and see where it takes me, really.

This captures the ambivalence and contingency involved in self-funding decisions, showing that this is not necessarily the activity of the overly optimistic or naïve.

Advocacy for access to personalised cancer medicines as part of NHS care takes on different forms and is not solely the preserve of patients. One advocate, Michelle, had a background in public relations and a high profile on social media and had been spurred into action by the death of a parent who had not been able to access targeted therapies as soon as she had hoped, as she explains in the quote below:

> it'd taken me a year [to win the appeal], and it was literally a year before I, you know, that I'd found it and then it had taken a year to do it, so she was virtually in a hospice by the time we, we got this damn drug approved.

... however, she took it, and ... she lived, you know, and for her it was like, a victory anyway, it did extend her life, it did help her quality of life, but of course it was too late for her. So, it was important then to keep going. So I did about seventy Exceptional Case appeals; within the first six months after mum's death, and overturned all of those, so there was a whole raft of cases, and that was all over the country, from Wales and England, and Scotland.

Michelle's story is interesting because it speaks further to the creation of a new kind of expertise emerging in this area – expertise in challenging NHS funding decision making and advocating for targeted therapies for patients on a case-by-case basis. Michelle takes on cases and supports patients to challenge refusals of drugs by local Clinical Commissioning Groups within the NHS, operating in the absence of definitive approvals by NICE for a growing list of experimental treatments, as well as challenging the 'postcode lottery' between the different regions of the UK. She describes her work thus:

by the time they get to me, nobody's listening to them ... every avenue is shut to them. Nobody gives them an answer, and I think the most important thing that I do with patients, I've actually just got an email this morning about a patient saying, 'if you hadn't have empowered me, I'd have never have questioned' ... the first thing I do with a patient is, number one, I listen, I just let them tell their story without interrupting; and say everything that they feel they never get the chance to say.

And then, I say, 'right let's unpick it, and let's take control of it and let's see how we can help', and I think, many, many of them, I would say are in crisis by the time they get to me ... they're exhausted, they're devastated, they're weak, they're frightened, and [this] has brought about another part of what I want changing – advocacy within the NHS – as soon as they speak to me, I would say nearly a hundred per cent say, that's the best time ... I've felt in the whole journey because it's for me, I focus on letting them feel a bit more in control and understanding the process, and understanding how it works; and the change that gives to a patient and their families is, is really quite miraculous. And to me, it is so easy, I can spend fifteen minutes with a patient and completely change their mind-set and their journey, and I'm appalled that that isn't available to them in the NHS.

Michelle was a self-styled 'warrior' for her patients, who told us how she struck fear into NHS managers and bureaucrats as she campaigned to get patients the treatments they needed. As part of this she sought to tell patients' stories and to celebrate their achievements and characteristics, rendering them popular as a means of garnering support for her efforts to get them what they need. Michelle posted links to blogs, posts and crowdfunding appeals by 'her patients' online and sought gifts from donors to surprise them on special occasions, such as tickets to the theatre. She was funded by private donations and did not want to be too critical about the pharmaceutical companies or the NHS as a public institution. Michelle also expressed reservations about how quickly some patients sought crowdfunding, preferring to try to challenge the NHS first to secure treatment. In so doing she operated among the clash of evidence, expertise and values of public and private care, forging what she framed as a new expertise that was required to navigate their growing complexity in the genomic era.

The private patient and advocacy stories we have explored here are, of course, just a small fraction of the kinds of experiences patients faced with difficult decisions around targeted treatments they had to navigate in the course of their cancer. We have shown how being a private patient is not about being filled with hope or optimism, but is marked by ambivalence, including feelings of guilt and obligations to other patients that must be managed, sometimes in public and sometimes very much in private. We have also shown how these dynamics open up new kinds of biosocial collectives around subtypes and drugs sought, and roles for patients and their supporters as advocates and other kinds of experts in personalised cancer medicine. Yet we also have to appreciate that these kinds of activities are being enacted by, and reinforcing the cultural capital of, a relatively exclusive kind of patient and advocate – often younger professionals who are articulate and tech-savvy, able to use social media to good effect to explore their experiences and connect with others. These already privileged patients and advocates are operating at the intersections of private medicine and social media, which further 'buttresses their sense of personal action, freedom and responsibility' (Van Dijck and Poell 2013: 10) as they access these treatments for themselves and others in an effort to extend their and others' futures. At the same time, they enact critical interventions in public space, challenging what they frame as the failures and inequities of the NHS. But this is not presented as an attack on the foundations of a public service. Instead, critique is offered in the spirit of improving the NHS, as private and public forms of medicine are inevitably entangled therein.

Crowdfunding: crafting futures in the digital economy

These entanglements of private and public care and privileged kinds of identities are particularly apparent in the arena of crowdfunding for cancer treatments. A *British Medical Journal* study reports that there has been a significant increase in online crowdfunding for alternative treatments on platforms such as GoFundMe and Just Giving, suggesting that, since 2012, £8 million has been raised, mostly for treatments in clinics abroad.[8] Other patients are fundraising for experimental treatments not available on the NHS, including targeted therapies. A recent BBC report found that £20 million was raised on crowdfunding sites between February 2018 and 2019 for cancer treatments not available on the NHS.[9] Clinics providing these treatments abroad also combine alternative and experimental treatments, and there is confusion about what kinds of treatments are showing positive effects in media reporting on so-called 'miracle cures'. For example, a recent *Daily Mirror* article[10] on a 'terminally ill mum' who had received successful 'alternative care' at a clinic in Mexico was publicly criticised by an oncologist for not making it clear that Alectinib, a targeted treatment for a subtype of lung cancer (ALK positive), was probably responsible for this woman's good outcome, rather than alternative therapies such as the coffee enemas featured in the article.[11] The press has a central role in creating a profile for fundraisers as well as criticising the dangers of 'quackery' in this arena. As the *BMJ* notes, 'Newspaper and TV reports on people with cancer drive donors to the crowdfunding sites, sometimes attracting the attention of celebrities, who boost funds. They also encourage others to seek the same treatment.'[12]

In this section, we will look more closely at the activities and experiences of cancer patients fundraising online for targeted therapies to explore what new kinds of cancer identities, work and public–private arrangements are developing as these sites proliferate. To understand how financial and cultural value is created by these practices we will draw on scholarship about digital capitalism which seeks to trace how value is accrued and by whom. This means we need to examine not just the efforts of fundraisers but of the platforms that host their activities, and the ways in which these are shared across other social media platforms and mainstream media through processes of cross-syndication which entwine social and mass media logics (Van Dijck and Poell 2013). We will also consider how fundraising becomes successful and what kinds of qualities and attributes fundraisers need to cultivate in order to be effectual. As Steinberg (2015) has argued, 'survivorship' has replaced 'victimhood' as a key subjectivity of 'good' cancer patienthood, and social media invites audiences to form judgements about the qualities and worth of the cancer patients seeking their help. Exploring how some fundraisers work to become popular to generate funds, we consider an array of other kinds of activities beyond raising money, such as being profiled in local media, blogging, undertaking charitable work and producing different cultural outputs such as books and art. We consider how fundraisers turn themselves into brands and establish popularity through the use of metrics that are key to the functioning of the social media platforms. Being a worthy investment is key to success with fundraising, but how does this happen, and how does it feel to those involved in doing this kind of work?

Crowdfunding sites are by now a familiar feature of life online. Many of us will have donated to fundraising efforts by family and friends, and perhaps we have also donated to strangers when their stories touch us. Seeking donations for cancer therapies online is typically driven by a sense of necessity as someone's cancer progresses and options for treatment narrow. Fundraising sites are often run by family or friends rather than the patient directly, but patients nevertheless play an important role as the 'face' of the campaign, and this includes providing often quite intimate details about their hopes and aspirations, as well as their experiences of treatment, in a series of updates and links to blogs, Facebook pages and other social media posts. Analysing a set of 15 fundraising campaigns for personalised cancer medicine identified via online searches of the main crowdfunding platforms, we can identify a particular set of discourses or tropes about the worthiness of the cancer patient seeking treatment which point to their admirable qualities, caring responsibilities and track record/commitment to 'giving back' to the community through fundraising and campaigning for charities and worthy causes. As Stage (2017) has shown, being positive, aspirational, determined, grateful, funny, entertaining and caring are important in cancer blogging. Positivity is also important to successful fundraising, but so too is being a good parent or partner and a skilled worker or artisan. Gratitude to all of the donors, large and small, whether through direct donations or through organising discos, cake stalls or sponsored walks, is also vital.

One crowdfunder, Claire, whose posts we followed until her death from secondary breast cancer, skilfully combined these various discourses across her fundraising, blog and Facebook pages. Claire's initial fundraising effort raised £15k over 17 months for targeted treatments not available on the NHS, and she moved to a different platform shortly before her death because the first platform had been taken over by another site and no longer supported PayPal payments for personal fundraising. Claire noted that at this point she had not had to use the money for the drugs, but that there was still a need to raise further money because treatments might be available soon and they are very expensive. Claire's fundraising site was mainly shared through her Facebook page, various campaigns she supported, and press coverage that she attracted. The Facebook page includes posts that celebrated the numbers of likes and shares her page achieved and asked people to donate on key occasions such as 'Giving Tuesday'. The page includes links to her blog, which tells Claire's story of living with secondary breast cancer over a number of years, and is heavily focused on her desire to give her teenage child a normal life and her sense of guilt that this will not be possible. There are a lot of images on the blog of Claire and her child smiling together in their home, on holiday and at various events, which are reshared on the fundraising site and Facebook. Claire tells the story of having to give up a professional job to become a full-time cancer patient, recounting the ups and downs of treatments and results, describing her hopes and gratitude, disappointments and frustrations. Her story includes details of her campaigning work with a breast cancer charity and campaign group for access to targeted treatments, with numerous links to press articles, profiles and TV news features. Although she provides some information about the specific molecular profile of her cancer and the kinds of drugs she needs, her profile pitches cancer as a disease that affects everyone. She shares humorous details of living with cancer every day and stresses the importance of taking pleasure in the little things, like getting a new haircut. Combining these different registers and sharing content across these different digital platforms allowed Claire to build up a profile as a worthy investment herself, in part by creating a space where criticism of the need to do this work is articulated. Through these accounts Claire constructed her online identity as both ordinary and exceptional. She is at once thrust into the world of cancer care and politics, but she is also just like you and me, wanting to do the best for our families. The final post about Claire's death, by her family, pays tribute to her campaigning work.

For other crowdfunders, being an advanced cancer patient seeking targeted treatments not available on the NHS has opened up new vistas of cultural work as author, poet or artist. Tom was a successful artist prior to his diagnosis with advanced cancer, but his efforts to access targeted treatment on the NHS were unsuccessful, so his partner turned to crowdfunding. The fundraising campaign has been very successful, trending on the crowdfunding platform at one point, and raising over £200k in less than 30 months. The site and related posts and pages by Tom, as well as media coverage of his plight, are replete with emotions of gratitude, anger and hope. But they all start from the position that Tom is a loving husband and father and a successful and much-loved public figure with considerable cultural capital who has entered into an intense period of creativity as he faces up to his illness. In one broadsheet newspaper article about Tom, his story is recounted as one of success, followed by pain and despair and then a new life of art and privately funded treatments supported by online fundraising. Tom's reluctance to seek funding this way, and his anger at underfunding of the NHS, pepper the accounts of his situation, as do his struggles to produce art, remain positive and inspire others. Art, politics and science feature in his personal story and engagement with public issues. The fundraising page is somewhat off-centre from these activities, not always mentioned or linked to, but nevertheless crucial to the way in which Tom is managing his condition. The site itself is managed by his partner, and this involves updates which include an emotionally charged video where his partner speaks about her family's hope for the treatment, as well as her exhaustion and gratitude. It includes poignant stories about people who are themselves facing difficult situations or do not have a great deal of money, such as a child who had lost a parent to cancer, who have donated to Tom's treatment. In the midst of these emotive stories we find links to bank account information, but there are few details about what the money buys in the way of treatment; rather there is a sense that options are being held open should Tom choose to pursue alternative therapies or other treatments using the funds raised.

We also identified more overt appeals for funds by other public patients such as Gillian, who has advanced ovarian cancer. It is interesting to note, however, that this fundraising effort was not as successful as that of other crowdfunders in our study. Gillian raised just short of £25k in 14 months. Although this was not for a particular targeted treatment, it was organised around the prospect of needing such treatment in the future and, as with other fundraisers, it included the possibility of funds being used for alternative as well as targeted therapies. We were fortunate to be able to interview Gillian before her health deteriorated and as her fundraising initiative was launched. Many of the themes in her voluminous social media posts and media coverage are present in her interview. Like all of the crowdfunders we have followed, Gillian is a young woman who was diagnosed after a diagnostic odyssey of missed symptoms and near death, in her case with late-stage cancer of the ovaries. Gillian's story is of a life that has fundamentally changed following her diagnosis, not just because of the extensive surgery and treatment regimes she has had to undertake, but because she has made being a cancer patient a full-time job. She has become an author and her books have achieved modest success in what is a busy market of cancer biographies and self-help books. Prior to setting up her crowdfunding page, Gillian was already deriving financial value from her cancer patienthood via her books and work as an alternative therapist and teacher.

Gillian has created a complex web of outputs and activities designed to inspire other patients, often based around memes or quotes that she thinks are particularly positive and upbeat. In her interview she told us about one of these:

> I saw a quote the other day which I really liked and it was 'did you have a bad day or a bad ten minutes you milked all day?' and I think that's so true, people focus on the negatives all of the time and people

are martyrs ... a lot of people say to me 'oh you must be so down all the time, you must cry a lot?' and I'm like 'why must I?', it's just about enjoying life.

This theme of resilience is further underscored by Gillian's use of language from youth culture, when she refers to her supporters and followers as 'bitches' or 'motherfucking warriors' and tags her posts with hashtags such as 'StillHereBitches'. At the same time, Gillian told us she 'hates it' when people say they have 'lost the fight with cancer': 'I absolutely loathe any battle survivor victim fight terminology', because cancer is not the enemy but 'part of me'. This captures the cacophony of competing emotions and aspirations that feature in this public version of cancer patienthood, reflecting the contradictory position that patients find themselves in, where they aspire to high-quality targeted treatment personalised to them but fear that it will not work in the end. One way of managing this for Gillian is to appeal to the ubiquity of cancer: 'we are all terminal; our life is precious'.

Gillian's investment in complementary therapy, as a recipient and practitioner, is also mixed with her investment in high-tech therapies including targeted treatments. The personalisation she advocates and seeks is hybrid and fluid and her engagement with scientific expertise is as partial as it is complex. Gillian refers to targeted therapies as 'Western medicine' in her blog where she also writes about her experiences of being on drug trials alongside her alternative treatments and therapies such as crystal healing. Elsewhere the targeted therapy is positioned as a 'maintenance drug' which is a small part of her 'holistic treatment regime' or her 'daily protocol for life' (which she notes is detailed in her book).

Unlike some of the other crowdfunders we have followed, Gillian frequently refers to her fundraising, and her posts link to her fundraising page across her social media outputs. Her discussion of fundraising includes the typical mix of gratitude and reciprocity we have discussed above, but Gillian goes into more detail about how she has been spending the money raised as part of her efforts to provide fellow patients with a protocol for how to manage their cancer day by day. We learn from these posts that Gillian started off raising money for Avastin, but elsewhere she posts that she is not privately funding Avastin any longer, and has used money for, among other things, a shaman. Her story has moved on to a focus on using complementary therapies to extend her life so that she is well enough to access an immunotherapy trial, the next hope for miracle treatments in the world of personalised medicine.

Throughout these various accounts we can see the importance of being a worthy investment to successful fundraising for targeted therapies not otherwise available on the NHS, including the demonstration of expertise, being hardworking and aspirational, special, but ordinary, like you and me, and a good parent, partner and socially useful citizen. Being funny and likeable, interesting or provocative and thereby articulating the cancer patient's personality as a strong 'brand' is also important to success. Accounts are inconsistent and at times contradictory, articulating a fluid and complex set of affective repertoires of gratitude, regret, anger and hope expressed through sometimes quite intimate and emotive stories and images. These accounts are part of the 'like economy' (Gerlitz and Helmond 2013) that extends Facebook's network of counters, buttons and clicks across social media platforms which facilitate further donations and reach. Fundraisers use and build from their existing online and offline networks in cancer communities, alternative medicine, the arts and the media to further raise their profile and donations. Within this we see molecular profiles and therapies sit alongside alternative knowledge and therapies as people craft possible futures for themselves and their relatives.

When we turn to consider how this money is spent, we can see it supports private medicine providers and pharmaceutical companies who produce the targeted therapies, but it also supports alternative practitioners and therapies in some cases. What is less apparent is that these activities create profit for the social media platforms via fees, advertising and surplus value generated by the sale of user data (Zuboff 2019). But for fundraisers, producing these carefully curated stories of investable identities and managing how this value is derived and perceived by donors is not always easy or straightforward.

One of the crowdfunders we interviewed was particularly candid about her experiences and worries around these activities. Stacey discovered she had advanced breast cancer while she was pregnant, and, following the birth of her child, went on to receive surgery and chemotherapy. She was told at this point about drugs that might be good for targeting her kind of cancer in a further round of treatment by her oncologist, but she was also warned that these drugs were not funded in her part of the country. The oncologist suggested that she might want to consider fundraising. Although grateful to the clinician for the early warning, this caused worry and upset for Stacey, who was initially ambivalent about fundraising. Her family decided to fundraise on her behalf despite her reservations. Stacey told us how her family was already fundraising to support her, so increasing the scale of fundraising to cover drugs was the next step. Over the course of 30 months nearly £200k was raised by her fundraising campaign.

Stacey spoke about her enormous gratitude and the sense of being loved and cared for that came with this experience. But she also expressed ambivalence about their activities, which centred around worries about the burden of being a good recipient of support. Stacey found that as a result of the decision to fundraise on this scale, she had to research different crowdfunding sites and how to open a bank account for these types of funds. Stacey also found the work of managing all of the donations quite intense:

> It just went crazy and that is basically because, well, the fact my story was quite emotive and [where I live] there is still a very strong sense of community. Everybody knows everybody, and so immediately that I put it out there, it just … spread and everybody got involved … complete strangers were messaging me saying 'I'm gonna do this for your fund' … Snowdon, marathons … all sorts of crazy things.

The fundraising page and associated Facebook pages are filled with stories of the ups and downs of Stacey's diagnosis and treatment and her family life, alongside pictures, posts and gratitude for these various fundraising events. But Stacey told us she also found this 'overwhelming, in a bad way':

> There were maybe like three or four different events happening every weekend … and lots of people understood that I couldn't make it to all of them but some people felt I should be there. And it was really hard to say no to people who were raising money for me. It hit a point when I thought I cannot do this.

Stacey found the work of doing updates and thanking donors, as well as attending events and researching the best means of fundraising, exhausting alongside managing her illness and taking care of her young family. She also had to field inquiries from other cancer patients about how to be successful at fundraising. She spoke about how, in the midst of this 'fundraising whirlwind', she began to feel guilty that the money had not yet been spent on the drugs she was fundraising for (one of the drugs had subsequently become available on the NHS and she was not yet in need of the other drug). Stacey began to 'gently encourage people to donate elsewhere'. She also became concerned about what would happen to the money should she die – if it would result in tax on her estate. She spoke to the bank about whether or not it might be considered to be her savings and should be disclosed to the state, and renamed the account.

But the most striking part of Stacey's story is her worry that she would be judged by her donors if they became suspicious that she was not using the money as intended. She told us about a controversy in her online community related to one relatively wealthy family who had crowdfunded for a cancer patient who had subsequently died, and there were concerns that the money had been spent on nice holidays and material possessions. This caused Stacey to worry about how she would be judged when her family bought a new car, and meant the family chose not to spend their other savings on a motor home in case it caused scandal. Stacey commented:

> With these crowdfunding sites ... it's just a very grey area. I mean, is it your money? I'm not classing it as my money, but it is really ... I could spend it on anything I want to. It wouldn't be morally right, but I don't think it would be illegal ... but other people might not think like that ... So, I do think that crowdfunding is ... open ... to abuse from people who might not have the same kind of ... moral standard ... say you're raising it for treatment and you're now dead. Can [the fundraising platform] say 'Well, we're not using it for that now, so you can't use it for something else?' It's something that does definitely worry me because I don't want to put my family in that position where they're faced with any kind of criticism or open to any kind of questioning from anyone else.

This story reveals some of the hidden labour of crowdfunding for targeted treatments, including the emotional labour of managing obligations to friends, family and donors in what is a moral as well as a financial economy. Behind the carefully curated stories of positivity and hope as a solution to the despair and pain that comes as cancer progresses, there is anxiety and concern that also has to be managed as part of being a cancer patient and making private troubles public in order to extend their future. Entering a 'grey area' between charity and the market, patients are raising money for future and current treatments (and sometimes other things) *and* contributing to the profits of digital platforms. There is ambiguity, too, around how funds are spent, including by relatives once the patient has died. Some sites remain open after death and donations can still be made in some cases. Sometimes the family does not inform donors how money raised for treatments that were not accessed was spent. As with private patients whose treatments are covered by insurance or who are in a position to self-fund using savings, crowdfunders such as Stacey can also feel guilty about patients with less support. As Stacey comments,

> I'm fortunate enough to be in a position where I am able to write up my story in an articulate and ... logical manner. I knew what I needed to say and how to say it ... I don't mean in a manipulative way, but I tried to be clear and open ... so that people know what I'm fundraising for and why I'm doing it ... not everyone is in a position to be able to do that ... to express what they need and why ... I think that's really sad because again we're discriminating against people who need the help as much as anyone else ... So we are coming back to poor people being worse off which is depressing really because it's all becoming like a two-tier system ... it should be healthcare for all. That's the premise of the NHS and it's dividing people again.

We came across examples of these less successful fundraising campaigns in our study, such as a page set up on behalf of a mother with brain cancer, seeking funds to cover four cycles of targeted therapy, which had raised £20 of a target of just under £7k. There are no updates on the site and we could not find any media coverage or Facebook sites about this patient.

Stacey, like other crowdfunders in our study such as Claire, managed this sense of frustration and guilt about relative privilege by supporting campaigns directed at increasing access to targeted drugs which are focused on challenging the pricing policies of pharmaceutical companies rather than the NHS: 'It's not the fault of the NHS that they can't afford these drugs. They are being manipulated by drug companies.'

Conclusion

Some patients faced with a cancer diagnosis are turning to private healthcare, advocacy and fundraising initiatives online in order to access targeted therapies. This creates new biosocialities in and through the digital economy. Younger patients with later stage diagnosis of particular cancers who might share a particular mutation come together to seek access to particular drugs to extend their futures by a matter of years, sharing experiences and advocating for improved care and access to therapies. As part of this, they share experiences of private and NHS care, sometimes revealing and at other times masking their status as a private patient, and in so doing manage a complex set of feelings of privilege and guilt. For some patients and their supporters (for example, relatives of deceased patients who might become advocates on their behalf) this involves the cultivation of new expertise, particularly in advocacy and negotiating NHS bureaucracy, and/or encouraging patients to be active as their own advocates and self-carers. Experimental treatments and molecular profiling in the UK are part of these stories, but so too are alternative therapies and clinics or trials abroad. The NHS is lauded and criticised (alongside pharmaceutical companies). These collectives and new kinds of experts are not 'astroturfed' patient-groups (Largent et al. 2018), nor are they in the mould of traditional consumer-advocacy groups, but they operate at the intersections of public and private spheres and healthcare sectors.

Crowdfunding affords a particular kind of digital identity for cancer patients, marked by positivity, hope and intimacy around some of the details of their medical treatments and family lives. Successful fundraising involves cross-syndication, as fundraising efforts and stories need to be shared and liked on other platforms to intensify support. News media coverage in local papers and regional TV are also important in this kind of profile raising. Fundraising depends on capitalising on and extending patients' existing cultural capital to project an investable identity in the so-called 'like economy' of digital media. The production of these identities, compulsory expressions of gratitude, and management of the funds raised nevertheless requires considerable hidden emotional and administrative labour that can add to the burden on patients managing treatments and family life. This work produces donations but it also produces profit for the digital platforms that host these efforts, although this remains unacknowledged for the most part. Crowdfunding seems to be a popular option for patients who are already familiar with and engaged with cancer culture online, even before treatments are actually needed. Even after their death, crowdfunding patients remain as 'data phantoms' (Ebeling 2016) on some sites and pages, as exemplars for other patients who will inevitably follow in their footsteps. Through these practices we can see that cancer patients and their advocates are turning to the market for targeted therapies via the digital platforms of surveillance capitalism (Zuboff 2019) to craft a future for themselves in the face of a bleak prognosis and narrowing options on the NHS. An array of Facebook sites and groups, blogs, crowdfunding and other social media platforms support these future-crafting activities. An 'elective affinity' is thus forming between surveillance capitalism and expensive personalised cancer medicines in the molecular age.

Notes

1 www.england.nhs.UK/wp-content/uploads/2013/04/cdf-sop.pdf, p. 6 (accessed 20 June 2020); https://www.scottishmedicines.org.UK (accessed 20 June 2020).
2 www.news-medical.net/news/20120910/UK-public-oppose-cancer-drugs-fund-but-support-new-pricing-system-for-branded-medicines.aspx (accessed 20 June 2020).
3 www.dailymail.co.UK/news/article-6804865/Welsh-NHS-worker-denied-cancer-drug-shes-half-mile-England.html (accessed 20 June 2020).
4 www.cancerresearchUK.org/funding-for-researchers/research-features/2016-08-10-health-economics-the-cancer-drugs-cost-conundrum (accessed 20 June 2020).
5 https://www.theatlantic.com/health/archive/2019/03/drug-prices-high-cost-research-and-development/585253/ (accessed 20 June 2020); www.healthaffairs.org/do/10.1377/hblog20170307.059036/full/ (accessed 20 June 2020).
6 www.fiercepharma.com/pharma/roche-gets-nice-approval-for-breast-cancer-drug-kadcyla-after-years-battles (accessed 20 June 2020).
7 www.bmj.com/content/351/bmj.h3852 (accessed 20 June 2020).
8 https://doi.org/10.1136/bmj.k3829 (published 12 September 2018) (accessed 20 June 2020).

9   https://www.bbc.co.uk/programmes/p072q8sk (accessed 20 June 2020).

10 www.mirror.co.UK/news/UK-news/terminally-ill-mum-who-hid-14178690 (accessed 20 June 2020).

11 https://twitter.com/cpeedell/status/1110266603692851201 (accessed 3 April 2020).

12 https://doi.org/10.1136/bmj.k3829 (published 12 September 2018) (accessed 20 June 2020).

7

At the limits of participation

Throughout this book we have endeavoured to demonstrate the diversity, complexity and contingency of personalised cancer medicine in practice, focusing in particular on its meanings and implications for patients as they craft their individual and collective futures. We have encountered a range of ways in which personalised medicine does not meet the promise articulated in popular totemic versions of its transformative powers. We have also shown how its values and meanings multiply in practice, and the work that is involved in extracting or articulating this value by and for patients, even if it does not always result in effective treatments or cures. At the same time, we have explored how the value of personalised medicine endeavours, particularly larger-scale research initiatives, is linked to the future of the wider bioeconomy, focused on economic gain generated by providing better services for more patients. Across this landscape of value generation, patient participation is crucial – patients need to provide data, experiment with treatments and enact responsibilities, to be engaged and remain active in maximising their own and others' health. The development and mainstreaming of molecular diagnostics, monitoring and targeted treatments relies on patients to advocate, campaign, learn, test and tolerate tissue extraction and experimental approaches, for their own and others' benefit.

Participation is, however, not guaranteed and cannot be taken for granted. Publics and patients do not always participate as the P4 agendas of predictive, personalised, preventative, participatory medicine envisage or promote. Sometimes tests or treatment options are not available despite patients' or their relatives' or clinicians' efforts; at other times patients choose not to participate or are not invited to do so. Participation in research, tests or treatments can also be irrelevant or experienced as unwelcome for some patients, particularly those who have fewer physical, economic and cultural resources or are otherwise alienated from medical and scientific institutions. Practitioners mediate participation too, sometimes being less likely to facilitate participation when they do not see advantages for patients or services more generally. In these contexts, participation can be framed or experienced as a burden rather than an opportunity.

As Michael (2012) discusses, 'misbehaviours' among representatives, members of the public or research participants can encompass a range of ways of avoiding or declining participation, not all of which involve actively saying 'no'. Ignoring, avoiding, prevaricating, querying, challenging, deflecting, reworking and subverting can also be part of avoiding or resisting participation, as can silent refusal. Non-participation can arise from a lack of opportunity, inclination or capacity, as much as an actual refusal. Participation can also be restricted or mediated in practice, purposely or sometimes without planning, for example when someone becomes upset or tired. In other situations, non-participation is more overt, shaped by a politics of what Benjamin calls 'informed refusal' by 'those who attempt to resist technoscientific conscription' (2016: 967). Developing Rapp's work on 'moral pioneers' including 'refusers and draft resisters' who actively choose not to partake in tests in response to 'a highly complex, highly structured social nexus within which they negotiate and exercise personal choice' (Rapp 1998: 62), Benjamin asks us to consider how these acts of refusal offer a 'necessary critique of the assumptions and excesses of forms of belonging that rest so heavily on biological claims' (Benjamin 2016: 967).

This chimes with critical reflection in other STS and medical sociology research on public engagement with technoscience and biomedicine (see, for example, Horst and Irwin 2010; Degeling et al. 2015; Madden and Speed 2017). Michael's (2012) work asks what we are 'busy doing' as social researchers in this field when the participants 'misbehave'. Here, the parameters of engagement events are 'over-spilled' and in the process the constitution of identities, relevant agendas and technologies are troubled. Felt and Fochler (2010) have also argued that we need to attend to how participants 'resist' the framing of participatory exercises, including how they reconstitute individual and collective identities and salient issues and concerns. We take up these challenges to reflect on how participation was troubled through the process of our own research and engagement practices and in the genomic technologies and initiatives we studied. In this chapter we explore how non-participation and limited participation in interviews and observations unfolded over the course of our project as a means of critically interrogating the participatory impetus in personalised cancer medicine, offering this as a useful counterpoint to the stories of participation we have presented thus far, and extending our analysis of the threads of resistance we have identified.

We were inevitably limited in terms of the kinds of patients and other potential participants we were able to approach regarding our study because of research governance, including ethical approval to work in an NHS setting. There are well-known criticisms of the constraining effect of these arrangements on ethnographic research, but we will not rehearse these here (see Murphy and Dingwall 2007). Instead we will reflect on the implications of the day-to-day and micro-instances of refusal, reworking and delimiting participation that we encountered over the course of the research, starting at the beginning of our work when we sought to 'scope' the field.

Scoping personalised cancer medicine

When we began our project and prior to obtaining NHS ethical approval to enter the clinic to talk to patients in real time, we conducted a series of 'scoping' interviews with former patients and their relatives, in an effort to understand their experiences of and perspectives on personalised cancer medicine. We also established two Public and Patient Involvement groups to guide our research design, recruitment, ethical practice and dissemination activities. These participants were not recruited through the NHS. Although we gained valuable insights into the different meanings and challenges of personalised cancer medicine for patients through these activities, which guided our analytical approach in the research that followed, the participants who were most easily involved were typically white, middle-class and female.

Using snowballing and other recruitment strategies that relied on professional gatekeepers, patient advocates, charities and social media networks to recruit participants and representatives for our Public and Patient Involvement (PPI) panels captured a particular set of experiences and perspectives from patients, former patients and family members, who were often actively involved in efforts to control and manage their condition, be positive and contribute to research and treatment improvement – unlike other kinds of patients who were too unwell or alienated or otherwise disengaged from research and clinic care. Some of those who participated in our early scoping interviews or contributed to our PPI were nevertheless aware of their privilege, and made efforts to be reflective and to advocate for equality in the course of their encounters with our project. For example, some of the former patients we interviewed were involved in advocating for genomic medicine across various platforms, including in evidence groups in Europe, and as part of this they reflected on the (un)equal distribution of genomic medicine worldwide. One patient advocate, Toni, reflected on the extent to which this has the potential to exacerbate already existing health and social inequalities:

> So we haven't actually looked at personalised medicine, precision medicine, whichever you want to call it, nearly as much as what we'd like to. But, of course, it is going to be an issue. And part of the reason has also been that, in most countries with the highest level of deprivation, not only have they never heard of precision medicine or personalised medicine but they've absolutely no chance of having any access to it anyway … one of the problems of precision medicine is it's got everything going for it in terms of making the gap even greater between the richer and the poorer countries because these drugs, by definition, are much more expensive but they have a huge difference in their, of their potential impact. I mean, the instances of melanomas, for instance, has completely changed because of precision medicines and so, and gene therapy and so on, and, and all of the areas where there's absolutely no, no access to these things is the, in the low income countries.
>
> So … we reckon that precision medicines will actually make things worse, not better, when it comes to access. And, of course, what will also happen is, is that it will, it will make it much more difficult for people to even get the, what we would consider the very simplistic treatments because the emphasis will have shifted over towards the much more effective treatments.
>
> …

> They're very uncomfortable when I speak because most of the time
> it's all rampant, gung-ho, you know, isn't it fantastic type of thing,
> how are we going to get everybody … onto these medicines and so
> on, and then along comes [someone] and messes the whole thing up
> in talking about the inequalities that are going to increase because
> of it.

In elaborating concerns about the (re)production and exacerbation
of inequalities in access to healthcare worldwide and the implementation of genomic medicine, Toni challenged dominant tropes of promise
and precision, drawing attention to what Hall et al. have argued is
'the transition from industrial to financial capitalism in Europe'
which has effected 'deepening inequalities of income, health and
life chances within and between countries' (2014: 9).

Another patient advocate, Adele, who had survived melanoma
and secondary lung cancer, noted that an important part of her role
was to ensure that inequities were also attended to in terms of cancer
types, with patients who suffered from rarer cancers often neglected
by pharmaceutical companies and researchers:

> There's so many [cancer types] out there yeah, especially for example
> in ovarian cancer, high grade serous ovarian cancer is the most common,
> that's about 70%, but you've got low grade serous, you've got
> endometrioid ovarian cancer, now you've only got a small number
> of people but those are the folks who suffer cause there maybe aren't
> as many studies, because often clinicians will target the sub-types
> with the highest number. So part of my job as a patient is to say 'no,
> no, no, no we've got to make sure *everybody* is included, and it might
> be a smaller number of patients therefore the pharma companies
> might not be as interested but you've got to include them', so that
> was part of my battle the other day at a meeting saying 'no you've
> got to include these people' … Cause that was raised, 'why don't we
> just target the high grade?' 'No, what about those…?' … they could
> overhear this conversation and think 'we're just being dismissed'.

However, the capacity to challenge and tackle inequality from a
position of privilege risks further entrenching privileged voices, as
with professionals advocating on behalf of patients (including social
researchers). We can capture this by contrasting the account above
with those of other participants in this early phase of our project,
who told us how difficult it was to become involved in this kind of
advocacy or support work. We met Karin through a local lung

cancer support group. After an unexpected cancer diagnosis, only months after she had quit smoking, Karin started to volunteer at a cancer charity and then developed her role as more of a campaigner on cancer awareness and prevention. However, she found it difficult to attend meetings as she had to rely on public transport. Karin shared her experience of attending a medical conference to which patient advocates and representatives were invited:

> I've been to an odd one or two, [lung cancer patient meetings] and … to be quite honest, I don't know what they called it now. It was a little bit too sort of medical-wise for us. And we went with the impression that, you know, we've had cancer, can we put our point forward, and it, we never got to that stage … I can't really explain it. It was a little bit too technical, and all the groups that were there, they were groups, they weren't odd individuals like [lung cancer patient] and myself. So we felt a little bit out of place on that.
>
> … But the point is, the trouble is with that, doing these sort of meetings and conferences and what have you, it's the travelling for me, getting to somewhere.
>
> They'll say, oh there's a meeting at ten o'clock at [city in Yorkshire]. Now it's virtually impossible for me to get there that early. I know it isn't early in normal terms, but it is, to set off, I'm talking like seven o'clock in a morning to get a decent bus to get there, which you know, so it does put you off a little bit sometimes…

In addition to the structural barriers to participation and a feeling of being 'out of place' at meetings with professionals, participants also told us that online support groups were not always places where they felt and experienced support because the issues being discussed were not relevant to their day-to-day struggles. For example, John, who had experienced pancreatic cancer, told us that 'dealing with money' was much more difficult than the issues typically discussed in his support group, leading on to a long passage of reflection on these difficulties:

> dealing with money, that's one of the hardest things, benefits, nightmare.
>
> … I stopped work … for the last three years I've done about four months work maybe. Yes, I got sick pay, but that runs out … after twenty-four weeks … or … twenty-eight weeks, something like that … The forms they send you are ridiculous … the employment support allowance, sixty pages. I'm not joking sixty pages, and they, and they

want you to go back further ... than the tax people would go back. First mortgage and remortgage and all that. It's ridiculous.

They turned me down, turned me down ... because ... I hadn't earned enough national insurance in the last year. How could I if I wasn't working? Absolutely, it's like a kick in the teeth. It didn't make sense. How can they turn you down for something you can't – you're not in control of? ... I get PIP, so, so that's separate from the accounts, for the moment they can't do anything about that.

The day-to-day struggles of living with cancer, which included managing money and employment, and even the act of travelling to support groups, were readily discussed in interviews. Two pancreatic patients who were taking part in a world-leading trial involving genomic sequencing and novel combination therapies discussed the seemingly mundane issue of finding a parking space prior to their weekly clinic appointment in their interviews. One of these patients described the effort she made to arrive at the hospital early, to avoid the additional fees entailed in parking at a nearby hotel. This then impacted on research nurses' work patterns, as they continuously adapted to accommodate those patients who were arriving earlier than their scheduled appointments. Through these kinds of accounts, we come to see that genomics and personalised medicine research depend upon patients devoting time as well as financial resources to their participation.

The structural and cultural limitations placed on participation in cancer support and patient engagement were further underscored by the difficulties of discussing genomics and personalised cancer medicine across these earlier interviews. Participants could have very little to say about this area of medicine, not just because they did not think they had experienced it directly, but also because it was difficult to make sense of. Many expressed concerns that they were not sufficiently knowledgeable to have a view worth recording, or that it was simply not part of their 'zones of relevance' (Parsons and Atkinson 1992). These interviews were typically detailed personal stories of cancer journeys and anticipated futures, and genomics did not tend to figure for many patients. Sometimes when it was raised by the interviewer we found interviewees reworking the question to deliver information and perspectives of more relevance to them. For example, in one interview with Jane, a former breast cancer patient introduced in Chapter 1, who spoke about all of the research she had done as a patient, the following exchange took place:

> in a brutal way that is what they do, they cut you, they burn you and they poison you, in that sense, but it's got this nice friendly, you know, language around it.

> **This whole development in cancer research and treatment promised that we will do less of that by doing, by applying ... genomic knowledge. So, did you have chance to kind of read up that aspect of new developments in cancer treatment ...**

> Well sort of, but the, I mean the genomic knowledge is, for example ... I got eight out of eight for oestrogen and they tell you that, and then you go, 'hurray, I've got full marks', but you don't know what you've got full marks for, and it's, it reacts to oestrogen, and so therefore they can give you tamoxifen so it sounds like, you know, my personal cancer reacts to oestrogen and I, and I thought that's interesting, but that, I mean that's what tamoxifen's for, is to, you know, replace, or to stop the oestrogen being, being taken up. They also told me that I got eight out of eight for, what the other one beginning with P, progesterone, and I did ask, because I'd read a book by an American ... about ... dealing with the progesterone sorry, and they, they weren't interested in that at all. [But] when I said, so why do you test progesterone then, and they, they were sort of a bit [pause] they didn't really, I don't know, they didn't really, they didn't give me an answer ... I was particularly interested because this guy was ... tracing all sorts of things ... because I've had a lot of miscarriages and ... progesterone seemed to be, according to him, I mean he [was] quite a serious doctor, but he, he didn't agree with the standard ways of treating cancer; and I thought, well that's interesting, because I've had that ... but they didn't, they sort of didn't want to know...

In this account Jane worked the question about genomics into an account of her cancer subtype to make salient the story of her own research, and her difficulties with getting the treating clinicians to engage with her personal story and concerns about why she had developed this kind of cancer, focusing on the journey travelled rather than the future we asked her to speculate about.

Former patients agreed to be interviewed for a range of reasons, but a common theme was their desire to 'give something back' to the health service or other patients by helping with our research – anticipating a beneficial future. This reciprocity is, of course, key to participation in health and social research, and is actively encouraged in a lot of clinical research (although we were much more uncomfortable with being cast in this light, given that our research will not directly inform or improve clinical practice). In our study it also provided an occasion for participants to perform gratitude and responsible patienthood, crafting their own patient narrative as a process of recovery and reaffirmation after their cancer experiences. Questions about genomics could therefore become a kind of prop for the articulation of their own subjectivities, desires and priorities, as in the following excerpt from an interview with Carol, who had gone through two different cancers, malignant melanoma and breast cancer, one after another:

> **Have you heard about the 100,000 Genomes Project? What do you think the benefits and/or challenges might be of being involved in these kinds of studies from your experience of having cancer?**
>
> Well I think benefits obviously if people can be better informed that's great … the only problem with knowing is I think if you're more susceptible to cancer is you've got to live with that you know and it's how you cope with that really … day-to-day … some people are very frightened of cancer and … if they found out that they were more genetically susceptible then … it could rule their life. It's all about mind-set for me cancer is all about mind-set.
>
> **Can you elaborate on that a bit more?**
>
> Yeah because … I've trained as a hypnotherapist as well … I understand the importance of the power of the mind and I do think that … if you're terminally ill … you're not gonna be able to change things around but I think the quality of life that you have is determined by your mind-set and trying to stay as positive as possible for as long as you can.

This illustrates how participation was an active process, where the meaning of participation was reworked, including via subtle forms of non-engagement with the details of particular questions. This could include occasions when invitations to speculate about the future were reframed, in some cases to articulate more familiar and productive narratives demonstrating responsible and active patienthood.

Former patients and their relatives could also critically reflect on care received and the limited place of genomics as part of the wider future of cancer research and care. As we have said, this included situations where genomics was rarely touched upon. It also included participants 'talking back to science' by reflecting on particular barriers or challenges associated with accessing healthcare in the NHS that were marked by race, class and gender. One woman, Mina, who had lost her mother to cancer, told us about her uneven experience of care. Her mother, who she told us was a successful and independent woman and a manager in her workplace, spoke very little English, and so healthcare encounters did not always involve the kind of care the family expected:

> They [Macmillan nurses] didn't give any help because they couldn't speak the language. So there were no Asian nurses. So I thought hang on, in a place like [this] ... are you telling me that there's no Asian nurse who can actually speak to my mum?

Although elsewhere this participant praised the NHS and the care her mother received, her experience of not being 'fully part' of the care infrastructures around cancer were reflected in her account of research participation as not being something she would herself consider:

> I just hope they find a cure, full stop. Seriously I just hope they find a cure for it, sooner rather than later.
>
> That's it really ... that's the only thing I can say is just a cure isn't it? ... I think they did what they could have done ... they did provide support. Yes, we didn't take it ... for our own personal reasons ... let's say, if someone like myself went through it, I'd probably deal with it differently ... I'd probably take the support. I'd probably take the things ... try things out because I would know what's happening rather than not happening, and I would probably take an active interest in what's happening. So I think, um, information is very important.
>
> Do ... you ... try to take part in ... any way possible?
>
> No, no, actually no, no, I ... donate a bit here and there ... there's studies that are going on, but they've not yet cracked it yet, so I would have said –
>
> ... so you – you want to wait for the right moment?
>
> Yeah ... I'm waiting for the right moment ... Once they've cracked it, yes ... I'll be very interested then. At the moment, yes, 'we're researching on this' ... yeah, fine, alright, just get it. Just do it ...

there's nothing I can do. I'm not a scientist. I can't help them with that. They need to … find a cure. They've been at it for ages … I don't take any active interest in it…

This passage shows how the participant connected her experiences and capacity to take up care with active interest in information, in contrast to her mother, but did not go so far as to see this as invoking a reciprocal responsibility on her part to research, which was framed as something for scientists to 'get on with'.

Another woman, Saira, also spoke about the burden of caring for her mother, including giving up full-time work to look after her and attend appointments. When asked to reflect on the inclusion of patients in healthcare initiatives and genomic medicine, her account captures the institutionalised disconnection between 'science' and older black and ethnic minority cancer patients through a focus on language barriers:

> … nowadays more patients take part in not just trials as a trial participant but also take part in sort of designing research or how funding should be allocated and that sort of thing…

> Very difficult for black and ethnic minorities because my mum was – her first language wasn't English so she – she didn't even like attending appointments … Sometimes they're not in the right frame of mind to know what happened in – what sort of tests she had 5 years ago. I kept a track. In fact it was almost like a full-time job …That's a very big barrier for somebody who, firstly for somebody whose first language isn't English.

> So I was acting as an interpreter for her at all times. So she refused to go to an appointment even with another family member because she felt they didn't have all of the background information and she didn't remember any of it, and – and again, English was a barrier for her.

> So getting black and ethnic minorities on board is even harder because they don't see how, if they don't speak directly – and if you're not a direct participant and you're going through somebody else who's interpreting, it's not the same as having that direct contact sometimes. And I think it's really hard getting them on board.

Later in the interview Saira stressed the importance of communicating directly with BAME communities via spaces such as mosques in order to build relationships as a step towards improving inclusion and engagement; a means of co-production.

As Grace, a cancer charity representative, explained, building relationships was particularly important, given that interactions between the black community and health professionals were shaped by 'historically grounded' distrust over incidents such as the Tuskegee experiment.[1] She reflected that this has contributed to an under-representation of black and minority ethnic individuals in clinical trials, an issue which was also raised by Zoe, introduced in Chapter 2. This brought other kinds of additional work to some patients from ethnic minorities in engaging with the science. For example, when researching the Oncotype DX test, Zoe, a health professional, questioned whether she could 'rely' on the US-based TAILORx trial because of its study population, and thus looked to research originating in other continents for additional insight:

> There's a Japanese paper I looked at, because, you know, genes can be different, because all the study has been done on the Western population. You know, the Sparano [TAILORx] study, the whole Oncotype DX. So what's the relevance in a non-Western population? So a Japanese study has looked at it and … they've said there's no difference. So I said, I'm not Japanese, I'm not Western, I'm like, somewhere in the middle, I suppose, and it doesn't matter (laughs). Yeah, so it, it's genes, it's human genes, and, um, I suppose, ethnicity doesn't come into that, is how I looked at it.

Zoe's treatment decisions entailed an added layer of complexity as she reflected on the origin of study results and their applicability to her situation, issues not faced by the majority of our research participants.

Together, these examples of critical reflection about structural and cultural barriers to participation in cancer research and support, as well as instances where discussions were repurposed away from genomics to something more meaningful for participants, demonstrate the structural, ongoing ways in which certain voices and experiences are excluded from participation in social and genomic research. This highlights some of the reasons for the absence of less privileged patients and advocates from our research and from precision medicine more generally, pressing us to think more critically about the limits on participation in our study, as we now go on to discuss further.

Accessing personalised medicine participants

When we were negotiating access and recruitment of patients in the clinic, we encountered further complex dynamics of non- and reworked participation in our own research and the genomic technologies and research that we explored as potential or actual case studies. We were already constrained in the project design when we were only granted ethical approval to study specific genomic interventions in cancer clinics and to approach people who were interested in or had actually participated in genomic tests, treatments and research in order to prevent an undue burden being placed on those who had declined. This limited our capacity to understand why patients do not participate and further skewed our sample to patients with the resources to participate. This inevitably also resulted in our research only engaging with those patients in better health, as a common reason for non-participation, despite initial interest and even consent to contribute to genomic research, was that the patient was too ill to participate or passed away while we were recruiting for our research. Such constraints also led to a focus on particular kinds of cancers and not others. Although we tried to avoid concentrating on well-resourced and well-researched cancers such as breast cancer, this was the most appropriate area in which to study genomic profiling in mainstream practice, given its maturity in this patient population. We also focused on gynaecological cancers and lung cancers as less resourced and researched cancers, but this also skewed our sample towards a predominantly female population, given the focus on women's cancers and the difficulties we faced in accessing lung cancer patients who were very sick. This limited our insights into how men manage cancer and incorporate their understandings of genomic medicine and research therein (Wenger and Oliffe 2014). Our study of the 100,000 Genomes Project allowed us to focus on a range of other cancers too, but the dynamics of research interest and investment across different cancer types meant we tended not to access many patients with rarer forms of cancer.

Participation was further restricted through the recruitment process, as we relied upon gatekeepers to facilitate the projects. Clinicians' ambivalence about the meaning of genomics and personalised cancer medicine was a striking and somewhat unexpected feature of these arrangements. After working with a group of supportive clinicians and scientists to obtain ethical approval for ethnographic research in hospitals, we focused on particular case studies of personalised cancer medicine involving genomics. We approached a range of oncologists and pathologists working across cancer clinics and laboratories to develop our cases, but quickly learned that the focus of our study had little resonance or meaning for some of those we spoke with, to the extent that it was often difficult or impossible to organise their participation in the research or a role as a gatekeeper to other participants. One particular breast cancer consultant who helped in the early stages of our project development expressed some of this in an interview, where he was notably sceptical about personalised cancer medicine with a focus on genomic tests, treatments and research:

> I've been through ... a number of different fashions ... and also because in breast cancer we've had access to many of what I've seen as the potential roles of genomics in the future, we've actually been using this sort of information for many years. Now, the current obsession ... around ... the role of genetics and mutations changing life completely. As a breast cancer doctor ... we are lucky in having the two most important targeted, groups of targeted therapies in cancer by a million miles, tamoxifen and Herceptin.
>
> Tamoxifen, you do not test for genetic mutations; you check for expression. With Trastuzumab Herceptin, you do not test for mutations; you test for expression. So that puts me at the start ... as being in a sceptical position about the role of genetic mutations because the two most effective genetically based treatments are actually based upon expression, not mutation.

Clinicians' active non-participation in the promissory, transformative visions of genomics meant that accessing patients, tests and technologies to study could be difficult, as they were seen as insufficiently novel to be worthy of our (and clinicians' attention). Beyond a fairly small group of pioneers and enthusiasts for genomic research medicine in cancer who were keen to support our work, there were other clinicians who were much more sceptical about the value of genomics and research into its implications.

Other clinicians were reticent or frustrated in their efforts to participate or facilitate patient participation in genomic medicine and our study because of a range of factors. This could arise because the study or trial we wanted to follow was not yet recruiting or because there were concerns about the lack of progress in the initiatives we wanted to explore, for example when not many patients were being recruited and the trial or study was seen as precarious and in danger of failure (as discussed in Chapter 4). At other times, concerns about the burden of participation on patients or staff meant that we were not able to observe or approach patients for interviews – their situation was too difficult to warrant such an intrusion. These considerations were heavily shaped by the perspective of research nurses who acted as principal gatekeepers, but also our own sense of what would be intrusive, based on our research and personal experiences. As a team we constantly reviewed our ethical approaches, but also reflected on our 'personal ethics', which similarly regulated the participants we (re)approached. For example, in our work with pancreatic cancer, associated with poorer survival outcomes than many other cancers, of four patients being followed up in a particular study arm we were hoping to observe, two participated in our study. In one case, after the researcher approached the patient for interview in line with ethical approval, the research nurse disclosed that the patient had not received the scan results she had hoped for. At this stage, having gained the patient's contact details, follow-up became solely at the discretion of the researcher. In this, as in other instances, researchers became their own ethical gatekeepers; reflecting on how many times to make contact, what this contact might be, and when to stop. In this case, due to the sensitivity of the patient's situation, only one (unsuccessful) attempt at contact was made. This patient's experiences of pancreatic cancer trial participation, which are seldom recorded in social research, were therefore not included in our study. Such decisions surrounding recruitment were personal and contextual due to the rapidly changing nature of individual patients' health status and circumstances.

At other times participation was not possible because clinics were busy, appointments were missed or clinicians were too preoccupied with other, more urgent issues. We were advised to avoid relying on consultants as gatekeepers, limiting their participation and intensifying that of nurses, as in the fieldnote below: 'The consultant explained that it may be best to approach patients at the point of consent and to leave consultants out of the situation, "take the

consultants out of the equation because we forget".' This capacity
to forget also extended to recruitment for the studies we sought to
follow, as captured in the fieldnote below:

> Due to observe two patients – pre-assessment appointments at 11.20am
> and clinic at 2.30pm. On the morning of 05/06/17, I received an
> email from one of the research nurses to inform me that they would
> ring me once the patient had finished pre-assessment to let me know
> when to make my way to the clinic (the research nurses see the patient
> for 100,000 Genomes Project after the pre-assessment checks – up
> to 1.5 hours after their appointment time). Unfortunately, the research
> nurse phoned at 12.30pm to inform me that the clinician in pre-
> assessment had failed to contact the research nurse and the patient
> had been sent home. The nurse was frustrated at the miscommunication
> as they're unsure when they can next approach the patient – may
> have to be on the day of surgery. The nurse also informed me that I
> couldn't observe the 2.30pm patient – disease has metastasised. The
> nurse was very apologetic and agreed to inform me of any other
> patients booked in that week.

Sometimes clinicians' inattention or lack of facilitation was a more
active refusal, albeit from a position of privilege, as in this excerpt:

> As we were all standing around in the corridor the research nurse
> explained that they often 'stand around on one leg' between appoint-
> ments in case they miss the patient. Each week [clinical trials assistant]
> double checks with each consultant whether she can recruit the patients
> she's identified as being suitable for SMP2. She checks with [consultant
> oncologist 5] who seems reluctant to discuss 'I thought the Matrix
> had finished' 'it's not you again'.

These excerpts capture the emotional and articulation work of
practitioners involved in recruiting participants to our study. It shows
clinicians acting to protect patients and prioritise current care over
research which might bring benefits in the future, the 'waiting around'
involved, and the missed opportunities for recruitment, as well as
the complexities of dealing with busy clinicians and very sick patients.
Genomic research in this context was not standardised or routinised
in the clinic, nor was it special enough to warrant practitioners'
strong investment in studies of its effects or potential, constituting
another requirement in a long list of considerations for practitioners
to negotiate backstage and at times frontstage with patients. We

experienced similar tensions around observations in some laboratories that were under pressure in terms of workload and resources, particularly histopathology, where there was a sense that genomic testing was adding additional work without additional support, that its promise was overblown and exaggerated, and that our presence would have taken up too much time.

The make-up of clinical teams we worked with reflected gendered hierarchies in medicine: the majority of consultants were men (although the breast cancer team had a high number of female consultants in comparison to lung cancer, which had only two female consultants in the team) and the majority of nurses and clinical trials assistants who were involved in recruiting patients and caring for patients on trial were women. This stratification of medical work by gender accords with a long history of social science literature which demonstrates the feminisation of care work (Tronto 1993; see also Allen 2014; Allen and Hughes 2017). This work was intensified as nurses were called upon to act as gatekeepers and to aid with the recruitment to our study, given that consultants were often too time-pressured and tended to 'forget'.

Nurses took on much of the responsibility for the facilitation of our study in these challenging situations – crafting participation involved careful and intense articulation and emotional work across an ever-changing array of situations. This involved managing other clinicians' refusals and deflections, juggling staff shortages, training and workloads, but it also involved managing discomfort and a sense of concern about participation exposing deficiencies in the nurses' competencies or practice, as we noted in Chapter 5. Although we worked hard to avoid this and to limit the burdens created by our presence, we intensified and at times unsettled their work. This can be illustrated through our experiences of being told that nurses or clinical trials assistants were concerned about their level of knowledge about genomics and their capacity to participate in our research and enable the participation of patients in research more generally. For example, in one observation session, as we made our way to the clinic, the researcher asked the clinical trials assistant about observing other consent meetings for the 100,000 Genomes Project, and noted: 'she seemed quite reluctant to discuss this despite agreeing – changed the subject and exclaimed "you can watch me make a mess of the consent process and judge how I do it, yes!"'

Towards the end of the session the clinical trials assistant joked again about being observed:

> Whilst waiting around in the corridor [clinical trials assistant] turned to me and said, 'I bet I find out you're secretly judging how I consent (writing things down in your little book) – that actually you're a journalist (laughs)' – I tried to reassure her this definitely wasn't the case!

Here the clinical trials assistant expresses discomfort about the quality and implications of her participation and seeks reassurance from the researcher, further demonstrating a limit on participation we encountered across our research with practitioners and patients, but also troubling the identity of the researcher and challenging us to acknowledge the burdens we generate when we ask clinicians to facilitate our research.

As we have already noted, some cancers get more attention and resources than others, and some patients with particular kinds of cancers are more readily involved in genomic medicine than others as different kinds of privilege play out across research and clinical care. Patients, such as the advocate quoted at the beginning of the chapter, and clinicians can be acutely aware of these inequalities. A lack of privilege can be experienced as unwelcome forms of non-participation or exclusion from the promise and investment of genomic medicine. We have already explored some of this in the accounts of clinicians concerning patients feeling left behind or excluded from the possible benefits of personalised cancer medicine. Patients also discussed this, as in the extract below from an interview with a lung cancer patient, Hilary, and her daughter, Rose:

> [Rose] lung cancer's not as publicised as breast or…
>
> [Hilary] No, I don't believe, no.
>
> [Rose] …prostate…
>
> [Hilary] Prostate.
>
> [Rose] …even though it kills more people.
>
> **Yeah. What do you think about that? Why do you think that might be?**
>
> [Hilary] Because of…

[Rose] Because of the stigma with smoking.

[Hilary] ... the stigma of smoking. If I, if I got lung cancer, I'm letting everyone know that I've never been a smoker. If I got it, they'd be all sympathetic...

[Rose] Because she's not a smoker ... cos I'm not a smoker. So how've you got it? How've you got it?

[Hilary] It's like ... before I got cancer, if I heard somebody who had liver cancer...

[Rose] You'd think they were a drunk.

[Hilary] ... you automatically think of alcohol. Because, because we're not au fait yet on the environment, I don't think we're fully, fully aware of how the environment affects cancer, you know. Not just air pollution ... Stress, your working conditions, your living conditions ... they take that into account when it's your heart disease but they don't, I think, with cancers. There, there's a lot of environmental factors, not just what you've done to your body, 'cos as I say, people die of lung cancer who've never been a smoker or had any family members smoke...

[Rose] I mean, I work in [town] and there were a young lass over there who's actually taken a nurse to court because she was nineteen and she got diagnosed with lung cancer and the nurse turned round to her and said, 'Well, how many do you smoke, then?'

Gosh.

[Rose] And she'd never –

[Hilary] It's just an assumption.

[Rose] And it is just the stigma.

As well as discussing stigma and their sense of blame (see also Chapple et al. 2004), these interviewees implicitly criticised the focus on molecular rather than environmental factors in cancer, and highlighted the ways in which care providers as well as friends and family can make patients feel culpable and unworthy of support as they participate in care.

Accessing the experiences of working-class patients for whom cancers such as lung cancer were more prevalent was difficult given the extremely low survival rates of these patients. Although our sample consists predominantly of middle-class voices, there were numerous instances during interviews where concerns around inequality were raised or discussed, particularly in relation to patients having to seek financial assistance (particularly those in precarious work), lone parents, or people who had not gone through higher education. In one interview with Janet, a patient involved in the SMP2/Matrix study we followed, who we introduced in Chapter 4, these barriers to participation in support, care and research were starkly illustrated:

> you can go up to the [name of support centre] up the way, but they do it at silly times and 'cause I work, I … can't get to one, even if I wanted to … it's like me going to work and saying to my supervisor, 'Oh, I'm not coming in tomorrow 'cause I'm off blah, blah, blah.' I mean, she'd [have] hissy fits! I've got to come for treatment and see doctors [and she asks] 'Are you coming in?' Well, no. I mean, at first, I went, 'Oh yeah, no I'll be in,' and I thought why am I doing this to myself? You know, why am I sort of like getting down here, getting everything done and then running to get back to work? … I did work full days for a long time and then I can't remember which one of the treatments it was [it] didn't make me feel poorly but come the end of the week, I was just knackered; and I kept thinking, why am I doing this to myself. And I went in and I had three months off work 'cause I went down to the doctors, 'Can I have a sick note for a week?' and he sort of looked at things and he went, 'A week?' and I went, 'Yeah,' and he went, 'Why, what for?' I said, ''cause I'm – I said I'm so tired, come Friday.' I used to get home from work, have a coffee, maybe have something to eat and next thing I knew, it would be like Monday morning and I'd be thinking, where's the weekend gone? … so I went down to the doctors and said, 'Can I have a week off?' and he gave me like a month, and he said, 'Come back at the end of this.' And I went back and he went, 'Another one?' I went … 'No I want to go back again.' 'Take another month.' Then I took another month and when I went back then, I said, 'I don't want no more – don't give me no more, no more,' I said, 'I need to go back to work.' I was so bored at home … I think I actually needed that time off because when I went back, I thought I feel even better now.

Later, discussing her involvement in research, Janet expressed gratitude to medical science and willingness to 'be a guinea pig':

> I do take my hat off to all these … when they get all these samples in and they sit there and … whatever you do … That is just amazing.

I wouldn't be able to stop with everything (both laugh). You know, we need a guinea pig, [name of participant] I'll do it ... I will try anything ... they'd have to be ... really honest with me ... because the thought of them sort of thinking give her that, and then they're knowing when they're giving me it, then it's not going to [help]. That's the only bit what does scare me. Like if they said to me well we've got this, [name of participant] and we know for a fact it's going to do something. We're not 100 per cent sure what it's going to [do] – but we know it's not going to make it grow, and we know it's not going to make it spread, I'd go, 'Come on then, let's do it. When are we starting it? Are we doing it today? Well go and do it now.'

Yeah, because I've got to put my trust in the people [who] make that drug and I've got to put my trust in this place, and that, to me, that's a big thing ... putting your trust in somebody.

These excerpts illustrate the tension in participation for patients from underprivileged backgrounds negotiating stigma and a lack of the time and resources required to receive care, let alone participate in research, including something as basic as getting sick leave. At the same time they signal an enduring commitment to support research, to trust in institutions and companies and a willingness to be experimental subjects as a gamble on becoming well again.

Our study design, like that of the genomic technologies, research and trials we sought to follow and understand, relied on patients participating. But as we have discussed, this was hampered and reconfigured by the contexts in which we approached patients and the ways in which those discussions were repurposed by interviewees, for example to perform particular versions of good patienthood or experience therapeutic benefit. We also encountered numerous situations where patients were not able or willing to participate in our research either in general or throughout the course of interviews/observations, especially when we asked more specifically about genomics. Sometimes these forms of non- or reworked participation appeared planned or deliberate, but at other times they were more difficult or unexpected for patients, for example when they became very emotional or confused during an interview.

As we have already discussed, practitioners protected vulnerable patients from participation in our research and some of the research, trials, tests or treatments we were studying. This process of limiting participation was crucial to the ethical conduct of the research: the emotional work of the nurses involved can be seen in the following excerpt:

> I arrived at the nurses' office ... at approximately 2pm for the appointment at 2.20pm. We discussed the issue of consent and the nurse expressed her concern that the patient is very young and will be coming to the appointment concerned and anxious about diagnosis (too young to come through the bowel cancer screening programme). The nurse wasn't sure whether it would be appropriate for me to observe and to approach patients about participating at this stage of the pathway – better to observe pre-assessment clinics or those patients who have come through the screening programme. We walked over to the out-patient clinic building ... and made our way to the consultant's room. The nurse felt it was important that we checked with the consultant prior to the appointment about whether it would be appropriate for me to observe. I had spoken in the MDT meeting that morning and the consultant was in attendance – happy for me to observe.
>
> Sat in a side room away from the consultation room with the nurse – trolley filled with patients' notes – next to the waiting room. Clinics were running behind and the nurse kept having to check whether the patient had been called to the consultant's room. The nurse said they often did a lot of waiting around...
>
> The nurse is called into the consultant's office and I wait for approximately 30 minutes. The nurse decided not to call me into the appointment to observe as the patient had been given a diagnosis and was very emotional.
>
> I left the clinic at approximately 3.30pm and discussed with the nurse about our pathway for observation. She felt like she'd wasted my time but I stressed that it's important for us to attend clinic where they might be consenting patients regardless of whether they decide that it's not appropriate for us to observe.

Here the nurse facilitates non-participation in our research because of concerns about the health of the patient and the burden of being observed while being given a distressing diagnosis.

We can also see the complex work involved in the process of mediating participation in the following fieldnote:

> I met with the research nurse in their office ... at 1pm – discussed issue of consent and the pathway for the ... trial. We discussed the hopes and expectations attached to the SMP2 'don't even mention Matrix' because of the high failure rate ... [leads to] difficult conversations

with patients – feeling amongst patients that clinicians hold on to their results unnecessarily and question why it takes so long to see results...

First patient appointment at 1.20pm –

Sat and chatted with the two other research nurses about the possibility of observing patients through the SMP2 pathway – said this would be difficult as the percentage of people referred to Matrix is extremely low. She did however mention another biomarker test which might be of interest to us (is it a trial or standard care routine?) – need to follow this up with consultant. Unfortunately I didn't get to observe as the patient was struggling with chemo and the consultant decided it wouldn't be appropriate for the research nurse to approach the patient at this stage and seek consent to SMP2.

The next patient appointment wasn't until 3.40pm so ... typed up my notes ... I was attending on an unusually disruptive day – the research nurse doesn't usually go on the ward and the other clinic appointments were cancelled. The research nurse consented a patient to the 100k genome project (I asked if I could observe but she felt it wasn't appropriate – first time she'd consented) for a gynaecological cancer patient. The patient had been particularly unwell but really felt like they wanted to participate for the sake of others in the future.

This excerpt further illustrates how recruitment and participation took considerable choreography in the context of busy, often understaffed clinics where clinical teams are formed on each occasion the clinic convenes. Participation in personalised medicine was acutely difficult to deliver for sick and vulnerable patients facing foreshortened futures in this complex, pressurised environment.

On other occasions patients or their relatives declined to participate because they were too unwell or overwhelmed by their experiences, as in the fieldnote excerpt below:

While waiting for the specialist nurse, the couple sitting in the waiting area carefully reading the information sheet. The wife was still reading the information sheet when her husband questioned her very quietly. I could see ... that he was pointing out the end of the consent form. The wife carried on reading the information sheet carefully. After several minutes, the husband then come over and told me that they won't consent for my observations. He said, 'If it was ingrown toenail, she would do anything but it has been so traumatic' and he awkwardly smiled. Then he said, they both have educational background and appreciate the value of research. But he said participating in 100,000 Genomes Project was enough and wanted her to focus on recovery.

This 'informed refusal' (Benjamin 2016) captures some of the burdens of participation in research, given that patients were often approached about research studies in the course of difficult and sometimes overwhelming treatment protocols. We can also identify some of this burden by reflecting on instances where patients initially agreed to participate but then did not respond to follow-up enquiries. At other times they did not attend appointments where their consent was being sought to participate in genomic research (and our research). This non-attendance was a common occurrence and can be explained in part by the complexities of the research recruitment arrangements and the requirement of patients to attend yet another appointment which could be quite lengthy. However, we might also think about non-attendance as a means of troubling or reworking the salience of our focus on genomics as special and of experiences of genomic studies as particularly worthy of social research – in this case the patient's relative explained quite clearly it is simply not important enough to justify time and energy that is already in short supply.

Given how sick and how busy patients are, it is remarkable that they find the time to participate in research that does not benefit them directly, including our study. Their participation did generate opportunities to reflect on identities and to express concerns, and to tell their stories more generally, but it also formed part of their responsibilities to reciprocate care or help future patients, including perhaps their own families. This kind of participation was not, however, without its limits, some of which could be quite discomforting for all involved. Misunderstandings about the purpose of our research, the role of the interviewer and the potential to benefit were among the most difficult aspects of these limits on participation. This is not because participation was somehow not 'up to par' as a result, but because it demonstrates some of the deep-rooted problems with the participatory logic of personalised medicine, which relies on a complex consent process to gather data but places considerable burdens on patients in terms of time and thinking through their participation, taking advantage of patients' need to reciprocate care and glossing over the benefit they might receive as a result. As we discussed in Chapter 5, patients can be inventive in obtaining value from participation despite these issues, eschewing the need to be genomically literate, for example. But this kind of revaluation also curtailed participation. We can illustrate this in the following excerpt from an interview with Terry, after her surgery for colorectal cancer, who was initially confused about the research she had participated in:

So I'm just going to ask you a little bit about the [research study].

Yes.

Yeah. Don't worry, no technical questions (laughs).

Gosh, yeah. Keep reading that information leaflet you gave me then.

... so how were you approached about it? Was it [research nurse] who approached you ...?

You know, no, things are very – getting very mixed up, cos I've seen so many people ... I know [research nurse] approached me, yeah, no, I ... so it wasn't you then, was it, initially?

No.

Because I know you came in on –

I was there on the day that you had the surgery.

Yeah, the surgery, that's it.

Yeah.

So obviously I'd been to – so it probably was [research nurse] then, I'm actually –

Don't worry about it.

Yeah, yeah, I'm sure ... because there was ... your study, [research nurse] study and there was this other study that I did as well ... and they were all – I think I must have been asked all on the same day, yeah, so it's probably [research nurse] that said about the genomes as well then. Yeah.

And what kind of shaped your decision around it? Was it an easy decision to say yes...

Well, I'm not being funny, but I think anything, when it's to do with research, if it's not sort of – not [going to] take up a lot of time, but it – you know, because obviously with everything else you've got going on, you know, with having what you've got, you've got cancer and that, you don't want something that's going to take [a long time] – cos … you're, you're focused on what's wrong with you … So … if it was a study that was gonna, say I've got to do like sort of filling in of this and filling in of that or, just, I probably wouldn't – might not have done it. But … when [research nurse] explained more or less that it wasn't too … time consuming and I didn't have to do loads of forms and that, yeah, I was quite willing to do it … I mean, this sort of thing could help somebody I know, my family, my grand-children further down the line, you know, that's how I look, look at things anyway …

Here Terry struggles to make sense of what she has agreed to be part of and our role therein, falling back on familiar logics of reciprocity, future benefit and active patienthood to justify her involvement and collaborating with the researcher, while masking the lack of engagement in or salience of genomics.

Public engagement

Our study did not just take place in hospitals and clinics; we also endeavoured to study how cancer patients and relatives engaged with personalised medicine beyond these institutions, through advocacy, engagement exercises and involvement initiatives. As we have already discussed, these situations are not places where everyone feels that they can belong, nor are they always easy to attend given other commitments and barriers. Like our own Public and Patient Involvement panels, these forms of engagement are more often taken up by white, middle-class participants.

Lack of representation of ethnic and other minorities in genomic datasets and engagement exercises has, of course, been an ongoing source of concern for practitioners and policymakers. Much of this is framed in terms of a historic lack of trust on the part of marginalised communities, alienated by a series of scandals and exploitations including biopiracy, experimentation and commercial exploitation of tissue without any effort towards benefit sharing (Hamilton 2008; TallBear 2013; Skloot 2017). Together with contemporary experiences of institutionalised racism, this means that Black, Asian, and minority ethnic (BAME) groups and other marginalised communities also have a history of lower rates of participation in screening and research into cancer more generally. However, as Benjamin (2016) notes, there is a danger in framing these instances and patterns of non-participation as problems of trust, when the problem is perceived as being located with the community rather than the institutions and professionals who have behaved in systematically untrustworthy ways. And there is continued reason to be wary of a biomedical economy intent on data maximisation when BAME patients can be further disempowered by being framed as an untapped resource. This links to a wider set of challenges to the colonial and racialised practices of biomedicine, which have been dominated by white, male standpoints, framed as a 'god's eye' view devoid of 'bias' (Haraway 1988), but ultimately shaped by the interests of these dominant groups in maintaining power and privilege. It is reflected in Public and Patient Involvement practices focused on solutions and health improvements but reproducing health inequalities by amplifying a narrow range of perspectives, experiences and interests in the process (de Freitas and Martin 2015; Madden and Speed 2017).

Broadening and diversifying participation in engagement and in genomic research more generally becomes part of policy and institutional practices around these initiatives. The 100,000 Genomes Project involved a range of initiatives to access 'harder to reach' communities, particularly potential BAME participants. In 2019 the Yorkshire and Humber Regional Genomics Service that was part of Genomics England worked with playwrights and actors to produce a play in collaboration with ethnic minority community groups to promote inclusion in genomic medicine via 'culturally sensitive' education.[2] The purpose of the play was also to address and ameliorate some of the concerns about biomedical innovation from within these communities. The play was described as follows on the Genomic Medicine Service website:

A play raising awareness of genomics and the impact of genetic disease that often runs unaware within families from Black and Minority Ethnic backgrounds...

Mixing humour, personal story and science, 'Jeans, whose Genes?' explores the specific concerns of harder to reach communities using the analogy of mobile telephone and internet technology to demonstrate life-changing or enhancing possibilities in scientific developments to improve healthcare.

The play is focused around a conversation between two neighbours in which the black British Caribbean character expresses doubts and concerns about genomic research and the British Indian neighbour is more positive and hopeful about its potential to 'ease suffering'. The issues raised, generated in discussion with people from these communities, include historic abuses and discrimination against black patients and research participants and ongoing scandals such as the Windrush affair, which involved people from the black community being deported despite having lived and worked in the UK for many years. The black character is, however, reassured by her neighbour that researchers, and science, are not racist and we 'have to start trusting at some point'.

We also encountered similar concerns when we approached people from these communities about involvement in our work, including particular criticism of the use of informed consent forms as off-putting and needlessly bureaucratic. We offered reassurance about the ethical intent of this approach but this was not always convincing. Reflecting on this focus on resolving 'distrust' therefore requires further exploration. As Benjamin notes,

> by constructing trust as a cultural trait that some groups have more or less of than others, such discursive practices lead those engaged in trust talk to overlook differences within purported ethnoracial groups, disregard similarities across groups, and most importantly, ignore the larger institutionalised structures of inequality in biomedicine and beyond. (2014: x)

Accessing the experiences of subjugated populations is critical to driving inclusive genomic medicine and yet requires a systematic restructuring of systems of white privilege within biomedicine more generally, including in our case ethical protocols, informed consent processes and forms of engagement. It is also important to note that efforts to promote genomic medicine have the potential to both strip science of its cultural conditions of production – 'science is not racist' – and reify the problematic idea that race and categories of race are biologically defined; a notion which circulated in observations when patients were recruited to genomic medicine, as we see in the observation notes with a CTA below.

> 'You know because we're mixing more with different races it might tell us about different genetics; it's going to be massive' (family member)

[race circulating here which hasn't been as explicit in other consultations]. 'I hope so ...'

Conclusion

Not participating at all, being unable, unwilling, uninvited or limited in capacity to engage are key features of patient and practitioner experiences of personalised medicine and the plethora of research on which it relies. This limits the kinds of data and value obtained from participation, as well as limiting the potential for harm to arise from too much or too intense participation. At the same time, it configures the futures crafted, voices and experiences of participation and associated care to those well enough or sufficiently motivated or enthusiastic to participate. Some of these dynamics intensify promissory and positive tropes and underplay negative experiences in the process. They privilege enthusiastic voices and framings which emphasise the novelty or neutrality of science and technology. But attending to non-participation allows us to reflect on how practitioners and patients can refuse, resist and subvert these kinds of anticipatory logics through silence, or by turning away from the future to ground reflection in the mundane realities of managing day-to-day, or in stories rooted in the past, and privileging other kinds of care as a way of reconstituting identity in cancer's wake.

Reflecting on these processes of non-participation or limited participation also highlights how some cancers and patients are better resourced in terms of treatment and support infrastructures as well as research opportunities. Capturing the experiences of other more marginalised cancers with lower survival rates and less research investment (see All Party Parliamentary Group on Cancer 2009) was difficult in our study, because genomic medicine is being implemented with most success in cancers with a track record of research and improved treatment and via well-established organisational infrastructures. This can map on to some kinds of privilege for patients; for example, breast cancer is an area with considerable research investment and improved prospects, and is also associated with visible activism and is more common among those living in advantaged circumstances. These confluences can mean that patients with these kinds of cancers, outcomes and backgrounds are more likely to participate in research and its associated care, including social research like our study, as part of their active patienthood, and to have more hopeful visions of the future. This further constrains the kinds of experiential accounts on which we can draw to understand the impact of personalised medicine, rendering less visible experiences of the dark side of care, including failure, ambivalence, despair, disengagement and rejection. Exploring the margins or limits of participation, whether deliberately imposed or arising from organisational complexities, invites us to think more carefully about the kinds of practitioners and patients who are not able to (fully) participate in the promise of personalised medicine, and the need to attenuate and challenge overly optimistic promissory visions to attend to these limits. It also challenges us to think critically about the responsibilities and expectations of participation in the P4 era, particularly the intensification of work for key practitioners such as nurses and for patients as well.

Notes

1 See www.cdc.gov/tuskegee/timeline.htm (accessed 20 June 2020).
2 www.genomicsengland.co.UK/understanding-genomics/jeans-whose-genes/ (accessed 15 October 2019).

Conclusion

Future-crafting

Personalised cancer medicine is developing unevenly across a range of tests, treatments and research initiatives. Traversing local and personal quests for care, together with global networks of services, research and innovation, molecular information and tailored treatments involve a complex array of opportunities and expectations, where access and success are stratified along multiple lines. Patienthood, value, big and little futures all multiply through these arrangements, but coalesce into specific, more common or acceptable repertoires of empowered, hopeful patients, prospective economic growth and valued national assets. The future of informed, optimistic, reassured patients, living longer with or beyond cancer by virtue of molecular monitoring and tailored treatments, is aligned with a vision for UK wealth and prosperity, and a health service leveraging assets to work for the benefit of all of its citizenry.

But alongside these optimistic, promissory scenarios, there are numerous stories of disappointment, disengagement and deflection where patients and their relatives do not experience molecular information as empowerment, or cannot access molecular monitoring, tailored treatments or trials offering experimental therapies. Practitioners, too, are engaged in a series of compromises and a complex choreography of care to tailor treatments and tests as best they can, while supporting research efforts now and for the future, in conditions of limited time and resources. Ambiguity surrounds the blurred boundaries between research and care, with each transition between caring for a patient in the present and thinking about patients in the future requiring moral reflection as well as organisation and logistics.

Through these activities, the future comes into the present, as Adam and Groves comment: 'the future is not simply beyond the present but is a latent and "living future" *within* it' (2011: 17). This makes the work of crafting futures a matter of living and working well, or as well as possible, in the here and now, while also thinking beyond this immediate horizon to future selves or others. The extent to which care for oneself and/or others in the present or future can be tolerated varies across time and across different kinds of settings and patients, with those with the lowest reserves of cultural and economic capital having much less time or capacity to care with or about genomics, given how little they themselves are cared for by society at large.

Our study of personalised cancer medicine exploring these different dimensions of genomic-driven research and care was designed to inquire about the work and value of these activities – who does what, who benefits, why? Within this we have sought to pay particular attention to how care and futurity operate, as forms of work and anticipation merge to produce cancer patienthood anew in the genomic era. We have documented an array of activities, discourses and expectations across our case studies, the sheer variety and complexity of which are difficult to summarise. Our impetus for summary is further blunted by our sense of discomfort about mining our data for academic capital in the form of new theories or concepts, given our questioning of these activities when it comes to molecular as opposed to social data. At the same time we owe it to our readership to return to our initial questions and reflect on how future-crafting operates, the kinds of work and value involved, and how we might rethink and revalue care and other work, value and futures, given what we have discovered. We organise these reflections into three main sections in this final chapter, exploring the work of future-crafting, its collective impetus and implications for identity and solidarities, and how value is produced and reconfigured in the process, before moving on to our final thoughts on revaluing research and care in personalised cancer medicine.

Crafting futures as care work in personalised cancer medicine

To care is to anticipate and tend to an uncertain future, to enable and enliven an ongoing identity and maintain a place in the world.

Care features prominently in feminist analyses of technoscience and biomedicine, drawing our conceptual and empirical attention to its constitutive and political dimensions (Puig de la Bellacasa 2012). As Adam and Groves have written:

> in caring for another, we attempt to judge what futures they project for themselves – what they want and need – and what they are becoming, both because of what they want and need and in spite of it. What we attend to is the unfolding potential of an individual and to what events will mean in the context of the fate we share with those we care about. (2011: 22–3)

Caring, like crafting, involves working with numerous materials, patterns, technologies, colleagues, friends, family. It can be relentless, at times rewarding, and at other times difficult and unpleasant; it can cause tensions and build rapport, involve misunderstandings, fractures and disputes, as well as new alliances, a sense of purpose and solidarity. Sometimes caring comes with a script, an acceptable way of operating; at other times it is a process of trial and error, working out, salvaging, seeking help and being open to doing things differently. Our work finds both well-established practices of care, of making do, alongside new forms, for example through social media and through the research/care interface. But care is often under-recognised and undervalued as work, left to undervalued actors or in between other activities, privatised and typically the preserve of women and lower-status workers or carers.

Our studies of personalised cancer medicine have encountered institutions and organisations at various levels of operation – from the 'high-level' government or scientific elite pronouncements of the genomics vanguard (Hilgartner 2017), policymakers such as NICE or Genomics England Ethics Advisory Group, to project leaders, principal investigators, patient advocates, through to practitioners operating in laboratories and clinics to deliver genomic medicine, and, of course, to patients themselves and their families. Across these dimensions we have seen a plethora of activities designed to institutionalise or embed genomic medicine in practice, through protocols, research initiatives, training and education. Each, in their own way, are forms of articulation work that invoke or deliver versions of care for particular kinds of institutions, individuals and materials. At one end of the spectrum, considerable emphasis has been placed on standardising and optimising partnerships across nations, institutions and public/private sectors, because of the prospects this offers for delivering better, more precise kinds of healthcare and economic prosperity, enacting care on a macro scale. This is complex and sometimes fraught work. But at a more local scale, caring is especially messy, involving everything from taking care in encounters with patients and colleagues to tending to the logistics of sample preparation, delivery and analysis, consent mechanisms, clinician behaviours, patient pathways and results interpretation.

Organisations and their actors are expected to innovate and be open to innovation through these various activities, which inculcate a 'can do' attitude premised on caring enough to be open to learning and change, crafting a more certain future, as well as inviting a range of articulation work to make processes flow and put patients at ease. Yet much of this work remains hidden and unrecognised, despite its vital contribution to the institutional transformations required to make genomic medicine work in practice. It takes place in the margins, between quantifiable activities such as numbers of patients diagnosed, recruited, surviving, and is often delivered by staff working in conditions of precarity – on short-term contracts or projects, in laboratories and clinics that are being reorganised, and in services facing staffing shortages. It happens in corridor conversations, phone calls out of hours, hastily arranged meetings and cobbled together solutions to problems as they arise. These neglected forms of care work for tissue, colleagues, institutions and, of course, patients are an enduring feature of the work of personalising cancer medicine, yet they remain largely hidden from view in official accounts of precision healthcare and research agendas.

Strongly aligned with these activities are the intricate practices of managing the emotions provoked and sustained by personalised cancer medicine, an activity in which patients and carers, together with practitioners, are deeply engaged. Cancer diagnosis, prognosis and treatment invokes a cacophony of emotions of fear, grief, loss, hope, stubbornness and stoicism, and personalised cancer medicine intensifies this rollercoaster ride across the rise and fall of emotions at key points of transition and opportunity. Caring for patients along this journey is difficult and ongoing work for carers and practitioners; it also involves work for patients who need to be seen to care enough about themselves and to continue to care for others around them, including imagined future patients, by not being too negative, ungrateful or demanding. Being careful about hoping too much also requires work from all of these parties, and this can be a source of tension about the benefits of personalised care, not just in the sense that hopes can be dashed, but when disappointments are avoided or discounted and care is experienced as absence or neglect. Working in these ways does not always deliver the kinds of outcomes or experiences patients or practitioners value or expect.

Experimentation is another key feature of the work of personalising cancer medicine. This, too, involves considerable care work for multiple actors. Even when tests or treatments are relatively well established, their uptake in practice is highly contingent on personal circumstances and expectations; their very novelty can be a source of reassurance and comfort for some, but, at other times, a generator of further doubts and anxiety. When tests and treatments are experienced as part of research, or sourced through private means or charitable giving, the idea of being on trial or on the cutting edge can give a sense of being cared for enough that one's future is worth investment, offering hope that is sustaining. But experimenting, by its very nature, is marked by frustrations, tinkering and uncertainties, and this demands particular kinds of care work to manage side-effects, maintain eligibility, source alternatives and cultivate a sense of control of uncertain futures. Here the work of being on experimental therapies involves care as a kind of risk taking, which inevitably means creating burdens for others who must bear witness or manage risks as a result of their obligations to patients or kin. Personalised cancer medicine intensifies this work by embedding research as part of care via the kinds of studies we have followed – adaptive trials, WGS and even smaller feasibility studies taking place locally. Tailoring that care to the particularities of individuals' DNA and that of their tumours demands work on the part of those individuals to maintain their sense of uniqueness and potentiality to remain on treatments and stay alive, and to support those who are ineligible for genomic and for other reasons.

This uncovers a particular kind of trouble with personalised cancer medicine that is inscribed into the heart of the endeavour. Knowing about cancer and its, and thereby your own, future in ever greater detail intensifies the care work of practitioners and patients, as well as their families. But knowing is not always welcome or reassuring;

it is seldom certain knowledge, it can make patients, practitioners and relatives feel hopeless and despairing, and it can undercut the moral and cultural obligation to be empowered through knowledge. Not being able to access a hoped-for treatment, or being told that one's risk is actually rather higher than had previously been thought, being too ill or otherwise ineligible to join a trial, waiting a long time for results or treatments that turn out to be unremarkable, or not ever finding out about that personalised genomic profile because results or samples 'failed' is not empowering, and requires an additional layer of repair work to keep going in the face of disappointments and setbacks. Improving genomic literacy is unlikely to be the empowering solution to these experiences, given their depth and complexity.

Attention and resistance to these intense logics of empowerment, progress and the promise of precision are, however, difficult to sustain. For the genomic vanguard, when practitioners adapt, query, ignore or forget as a means of mediating or moderating the drive for molecular personalisation in favour of more holistic notions of personalised care, such resistance can be a reason to accelerate transformation, education or reorganisation of their services. When patients are uncompliant or disengaged, their resistance can be dismissed, managed or explained away by relatives and care givers seeking more optimistic territory. Other patients sublimate their concerns and critiques to keep care givers onside, given that they do not want to alienate and risk restrictions on future care. Relatives, too, can end up silencing their disappointments and fears in favour of being supportive, optimistic, caring. Non-participation can be difficult to achieve or sustain in these circumstances.

This proliferation of care work underpins the design and delivery of personalised cancer medicine and its repercussions for patients, carers and practitioners beyond individual encounters with molecular information or tailored treatments. Care work is oriented around crafting and balancing liveable presents and possible futures, even when options are narrowing or eclipsed as results and treatments do not always bring relief or hope. Care work is also profoundly relational – a collective activity. As personalised cancer medicine develops, these collectives and identities are rearranging, as we now go on to discuss in more detail.

Crafting futures together

Our initial approach to answering the question of how personalised medicine for cancer is transforming what it means to be a patient was to foreground the experiences and accounts of patients, focusing on their identity stories, alliances, commitments, engagements and expectations. This was driven by a sense that much of the STS work in this area is focused on professional practice and activities. But as we interviewed and observed patient experiences, the role of practitioners and relatives in shaping and enacting these practices and accounts came to the fore too, and our focus necessarily shifted beyond patients to this wider nexus of care. This was not just because interviewing patients and speaking about genomics with them was difficult due to their vulnerabilities and other more pressing priorities (although this was often the case), nor was it a matter of prioritising more expert or authoritative voices in the face of confusion or resistance from patients. Instead, our more expansive focus came about because of the repeated experience of patients, relatives and practitioners crafting futures together, as a loosely collective and relational, rather than an individual, enterprise. We observed this across our research: in interviews where relatives attended and contributed alongside the patients who were participating, configuring the interview as a source of reassurance and an opportunity to reflect together on how things were going; in observations in clinics where practitioners, patients and relatives mulled over results, their implications or expectations and settled on a course of action together; in corridor conversations and other backstage arenas such as laboratories or team meetings where, although patients were not physically present, practitioners were actively keeping them in mind when deciding what to do next; on fundraising and other websites where patients' stories were narrated by and in relation to family, friends and wider publics. So we expanded our approach, focused on professionals as well as patients, and included the activities and accounts of relatives in our study, to better capture these dynamics of collective future-making.

Genomic medicine is complex, and practitioners often worried about patients', and sometimes their own, ability to grasp its meanings and implications for patients now and in the future. This did not, however, result in a 'top-down' paternalistic approach where consultants managed results and decided on treatment, but typically involved dialogue and sense making between a range of practitioners, patients and relatives as they tried to develop a shared understanding of priorities, expectations and opportunities. Even when patients were less engaged, more stoic and trusting, less interested in 'the numbers' or their subtype, personalising cancer medicine demanded that patients, relatives and practitioners collectively enacted therapeutic and diagnostic approaches tailored to patients' needs. For more active, involved, information-seeking patients, who are often younger, more educated and affluent, these collective activities might be more frequent and intense. Yet even for the most entrepreneurial patient, their experience of genomic medicine was always mediated by engagements with and between practitioners with whom they developed shared understandings and agendas as a means of navigating genomic complexities and opportunities. Of course, these relationships and shared understandings could break down, or involve tension and distrust which varies across time and place, but even when under strain the collective process of sense making remains. We emphasise this point to counter one of the most dominant registers of personalised cancer medicine: that of the empowered, individualised patient, making choices, sourcing opportunities, tailoring treatments, and of the power of genomic information in those processes. The patients we found in our research were doing all of these things, but never alone, always in collaboration, and in a way that was intimately shaped by their networks, relationships and encounters with professionals, family and friends all acting as care givers. Genomics was just one part of this wider story.

Reciprocity was a key dimension of these relationships: it occurred when patients and relatives obtained personalised care in real time or for the future; when they enacted gratitude for that care by participating in other kinds of research, charitable giving or campaigning on behalf of other patients; and when they sought to be likeable and accommodating in everyday encounters in clinics and beyond. Patients and relatives used interviews, clinic appointments, consent meetings and a range of participatory and representational activities as occasions to enact reciprocity, to tell their stories of more or less personalised care and its deficiencies within an overall narrative of deep gratitude and commitment to the NHS and its staff, and a desire to help future patients. Even private patients accessing personalised care that is not available on the NHS expressed their sense of gratitude towards it and their discomfort with not accessing care on the NHS; they worked to offset this through other kinds of campaigning activities. Alongside efforts to achieve or demonstrate reciprocity we also identified multiple instances of its absence, as patients, practitioners and relatives experienced ruptures or discomfort in relationships and shared understandings and agendas. Personalised cancer medicine, like other kinds of care, is not always attuned to people's feelings and needs, it is not always available as it should be, and it can be an additional burden or interruption to care which stretched reciprocity to breaking point, generating silence, disappointment and distress.

The collective experience and delivery of personalised cancer medicine has also seen the intensification of particular kinds of biosocial solidarities associated with entrepreneurship and novel kinds of expertise among patients and their supporters. Biosociality is typically associated with rare disease patient groups, working in close alliance with researchers, and, in the case of cancer in the genomic era, we might expect patients and their supporters to be formed into groupings around particular subtypes of cancer, perhaps even across cancers, where a shared mutation traverses these. Yet our research does not suggest that these arrangements are developing at pace; instead, we have identified numerous examples of patients forming tentative alliances around particular efforts to access tailored drugs, trials or tests, often based around the type and stage of their cancer, including its molecular profile. Lung cancer patients seeking access to trials of stratified medicine, late-stage breast cancer patients, ovarian cancer patients, and bowel cancer patients seeking drugs such as Avastin – all of these groups were engaging with molecular subtypes and targeted therapies, but not to the exclusion of others with different molecular subtypes. Instead, their alliances were premised on the struggle for more tailored information and options, and involved the navigation of the landscape of trials and approvals, charitable campaigns and NHS/private provision. They were often online, and therefore engagements could be episodic and fleeting, as well as more committed in the longer term, particularly for those supporting such activities, including families and those living 'beyond cancer'.

Entwined with these biosocial collectives we can also identify new kinds of expertise being developed by particularly entrepreneurial actors, combining public relations, counselling and support, politics, alliance formation and challenges to advocacy, charitable, professional, political, philanthropic, public sector and corporate actors. We are thinking here of the successful artists, authors, campaigners, advocates, fundraisers and spokespersons for personalised cancer medicine seeking better access to molecular tests and targeted treatments, often outside the NHS. These entrepreneurial experts are key actors in the personalised cancer medicine landscape – facilitating networks, multiplying patienthood and crafting new roles for their relatives which hybridise traditional 'advocacy' or 'consumer critic' roles, working across public and private sector agendas actively to craft futures for individual patients and their collectives.

Recrafting value

As we have endeavoured to show throughout this book, the promise of personalised cancer medicine is an enduring big future vision which can be found across policy and vanguard accounts of genomic medicine. It also finds its way into ordinary discourses in the clinic and elsewhere, holding a kind of totemic power that enables personal and collective futures to overcome cancer. Patients, relatives and professionals were far less interested in personalised medicine as a source of economic gain either for pharmaceutical companies or the life science economies of the nation. Apart from critical interventions around access to treatment (which, in any case, often focus on the failings of the state, not the profiteering of corporations), the economic value generated by personalised medicine tended to be opaque and disconnected from people's vision of its promise and their futures.

As authors such as Jain (2007) and Steinberg (2015) have emphasised, this economic value is inexorably dependent on cancer patients' capacity to experiment and take risks with their care in the hope of extending their life. In so doing it relies upon a broader moral economy where being a good patient means embracing suffering for the ephemeral goal of cure, as Steinberg notes: 'The willingness to undergo treatment's "cutting edge" takes on a talismanic power. What it promises to confer is not so much "freedom from cancer", as it does moral standing, a certain brand of cultural entitlement and recognition as an edifying subject' (Steinberg 2015: 130). Our case studies are replete with this kind of opaque exchange, as 'high-level' promissory discourses of economic benefit to the nation dissolve into affective repertoires and encounters of care loaded with pain, suffering and optimism, as together patients and their carers tried to craft worthy futures. For all their complexity and variety, these stories share a common pattern of emphasis on investable identities, working hard to be well, to be positive, grateful and determined.

Yet patterns – like recipes and other instruction manuals – can be hacked: repurposed, reworked, adapted and refined. This happens in patient encounters with personalised cancer medicine too: scripts could be resisted, other kinds of patienthood enacted and valorised, difficult questions and awkwardness laid bare, and opaque relations partially revealed. Through these practices new kinds of value emerged, among which care in the present took on a special value of its own.

We have discussed some of these reworkings across our case studies and in relation to our interview practices, where we encountered patients and participants refocusing attention on other aspects of their care beyond or instead of genomics, or resisting the burden of genomic literacy. Through these activities, patients and participants realised other kinds of value from their encounters with personalised medicine, gaining comfort and reassurance and bolstering their sense of self-worth in the process. One way in which this happened was by turning away from the future to the past, to tell their stories and reflect on their meanings and implications. This is, of course, common in cancer cultures, as Jain captures below:

> Trying 'to know what the past holds,' what alternatives and what necessities it contained, can become a near obsession for a person with advanced cancer faced with the slender pages of a medical report. Learning, for example, that cancer was there and went undetected in earlier tests, unannounced in earlier reports, turns the faulty reports into the material remnants of lost opportunities – of times when treatments may have been less invasive, more efficacious. Because cancer is always about time. (Jain 2007: 83)

Genomics adds an extra dimension to these ways of 'living in prognosis', prompting reflection on molecular subtypes, dormancy and mutation for some. But for others, the salience of genomics was overwhelmed by the process of reflection and remembering, where it faded into the background of complex narratives of lifestyle, heredity and environment. By resisting the urge to focus on molecular futures in favour of phenotypic pasts, participants decentred genomics and reworked the emphasis on ever more complexity and detailed information as a source of progress and cure. Personalised medicine reasserted itself as the holistic assessment of need and shared decision making: genomics was evanescent in that context, while nonetheless becoming embedded in our health services.

This disappearing of genomics also happened in other ways across our studies. We found it difficult to identify, follow and appreciate. Studies were sometimes delayed or faced difficulties recruiting; tests or treatments were not widely adopted or available; and it was not always clear that we were looking at genomics when we explored encounters with personalised cancer medicine involving molecular monitoring or associated targeted therapies. Practitioners as well as patients were unclear about this with us. Genomic results also had less purchase and salience than we might have expected, from patients ignoring the numbers, to practitioners nuancing interpretation, to missing or absent results. But genomics also disappeared into the background of professional activities and patient experiences more generally: it was not a core part of many of their jobs or concerns, it could be just another bit of information or test or treatment or research study for some patients, a vanity project, a doomed venture or a niche activity – for someone else, not for me, more hype than reality. Each act of ignoring, criticising or reframing recrafted the value of genomics, decentring it for patients and practitioners, refocusing attention on the meanings and benefits of care more generally.

At the same time, inequities, deficiencies and problems in delivering care were ever-present concerns for practitioners, relatives and patients. Caring requires time and resources and these were sometimes in short supply. So, in practices like reworking and reclaiming care in the consent meeting for research, patients and practitioners were inadvertently highlighting care's absence elsewhere. In squeezing in meetings, telephone discussions, consenting and training, in recrafting, and often minimising, expectations, practitioners and patients were highlighting the limited opportunities to care for the staff and patients on whose participation value-generation for the companies and institutions leading the genomic revolution depends. Patients', carers' and colleagues' expressions of gratitude and respect for each other for going beyond their contractual duties and obligations also highlight the absence of sustained institutional support in the form of time and resources for people at the genomic coalface.

Exaggerated promises of the value of personalised medicine to patients also came under strain in stories of delays, disappointment, ambivalence, irrelevance or failures of results or access across our case studies. This was most acute when it came to crowdfunders and other kinds of private patients seeking treatments beyond the NHS. Here a tension in the promise of genomic medicine was partially revealed – what good are all of these investments that patients and practitioners make in research studies, trials, experimentation with novel tests and personalisation of care if the tailored treatments that are subsequently developed are too expensive for health services and, therefore, for many patients to access them? Alongside formal evaluations of the clinical and economic value of these drugs, we can find a process of recrafting value among patients and some practitioners where the question of the worth of a life is uncomfortably apparent, and the immediate personal value of accessing the drug is such that patients and their supporters will go to considerable lengths to generate the funds required. These patients and their supporters take on emotional and digital work in the process, and experiment with treatments to generate personal value as well as further value for other patients who might access these drugs in the future by turning their experiences into a source of evidence and exemplar. In so doing, they also highlight, in passing, the inequities and exclusions of care and the absence of value for some patients. A notable absence from many of their reflections, however, was critical engagement with the political and economic arrangements through which drugs are developed and funded by and through the state working with the private sector. There was a tendency to blame the state, not the market, a lack of appetite for thinking about how profits are derived from patients and from public institutions funding research. Although a few patients raised this with us, it was notable how little scope there was to explore and question these arrangements.

Conclusion: revaluing research and care

We can draw inspiration from these and other stories of engagement, accommodation, resistance and tension across our research to try to 'imagine different ways of acting responsibly in creating futures' (Adam and Groves 2011: 17). In so doing we must resist the allure of standardising what Puig de la Bellacasa aptly calls 'the messiness of the present' and try not to dismiss things that do not fit with neat analyses and recommendations (Puig de la Bellacasa 2012: 203). At the same time, it is important to take care not to represent or speak for patients as a whole, and in so doing silence their differences and divisions, and to recognise that we must 'work for change *from where we are*' alongside our participants (Puig de la Bellacasa 2012: 210). In this concluding section we reflect on three opportunities for revaluing research and care in personalised cancer medicine.

At one level, our case studies of personalised cancer medicine are versions of the same story, which is that research can no longer be considered separate from cancer care; instead, it is intrinsic to the delivery and expectations of (health) care now and in the future. Cancer patients are experimental patients in the genomic era by default: even those outside of mainstream NHS services are experimenting with new treatments whether they are on trials or not. If we think of all genomic research in cancer as a form of care, and vice versa, then we need to reimagine what we are doing when we invite participation or consent or education and training for some patients but not others. We need to rethink the burden of consent and genomic literacy and the opportunities for care that follow from these encounters, following patients' lead, allowing our ideas about 'what care is' to be challenged and reworked in the process. Most importantly, this labour needs to be accounted for in how the benefits and challenges of genomic medicine are portrayed and audited.

Thinking of personalising cancer care as work is a political act; it draws attention to value creation, monetisation and extraction of molecular and clinical data, and invites us to ask what happened to those results and tests and drugs that were developed because of all that research – how are patients benefiting? It also invites us to think about the other workers, the nurses, scientists, doctors, counsellors, advocates, fundraisers and informal carers. How can they be supported to deliver personalised cancer medicine through care as well as research? Revealing the lengths that patients and family members go to to attend clinics, source opportunities, facilitate research, stay well enough to get and stay on a trial, be suitably educated and competent to participate, underlines questions about who benefits and who decides who benefits from personalised cancer medicine. Running counter to the individualising logic of personalisation, this asks us to think about solidarities between and among these different kinds of genomic workers, and how best to realise and share the fruits of their labour.

We can also draw on these stories of the messiness of people's experiences and differences of perspectives as a means to resist the allure of speculative mono-futures of entrepreneurial active patients, alongside many feminists and others within cancer advocacy movements. As Jain has written,

> Instead of focusing on hope, cure, and the survivor figure, elegiac politics yearns to account for loss, grief, betrayal, and the connections between economic profits, disease, and death in a culture that is affronted by mortality. If the term 'survivor' offers a politics steeped in an identity formation around cancer, 'living in prognosis' offers an uneasy alternative, one that inhabits contradiction, confusion, and betrayal. (2007: 90)

Our exploration of practices of molecular prognosis sharpens our elegiac politics and presses upon us the need to continue to account for and think about all the other kinds of experiences and subjectivities caught up in the politics and economics of personalised cancer medicine, including patients and communities who are silenced, or who actively refute or reject its possibilities and benefits. Being uneasy with this, bearing witness to contradiction, is a necessary condition of collective and individual future-crafting.

Bibliography

Abelson, J., and Collins, P. A. (2009). Media hyping and the 'Herceptin access story': an analysis of Canadian and UK newspaper coverage. *Healthcare Policy*, 4(3): e113.

Abraham, J. (1995). *Science, politics and the pharmaceutical industry: controversy and bias in drug regulation*. London: UCL Press.

Abraham, J. (2009). Partial progress: governing the pharmaceutical industry and the NHS, 1948–2008. *Journal of Health Politics, Policy and Law*, 34(6): 931–77.

Adam, B., and Groves, C. (2007). *Future matters: action, knowledge, ethics*. Leiden: Brill.

Adam, B., and Groves, C. (2011). Futures tended: care and future-oriented responsibility. *Bulletin of Science, Technology & Society*, 31(1): 17–27.

Adams, V., Murphy, M., and Clarke, A. (2009). Anticipation: technoscience, life, affect, temporality. *Subjectivity*, 28: 246–65.

Ali-Khan, S. E., Black, L., Palmour, N., Hallett, M. T., and Avard, D. (2015). Socio-ethical issues in personalized medicine: a systematic review of English language health technology assessments of gene expression profiling tests for breast cancer prognosis. *International Journal of Technology Assessment in Health Care*, 31(1–2): 36–50.

Allen, D. (2014). *The invisible work of nurses: hospitals, organisation and healthcare*. Abingdon: Routledge.

Allen, D., and Hughes, D. (2017). *Nursing and the division of labour in healthcare*. Basingstoke: Macmillan International Higher Education.

All Party Parliamentary Group on Cancer (2009). *Report of the All Party Parliamentary Group on Cancer's Inquiry into Inequalities in Cancer (MacMillan Cancer Support)*. London: All Party Parliamentary Group on Cancer.

Arnold, M., Rutherford, M. J., Bardot, A., Ferlay, J., Andersson, T. M. L., Myklebust, T. A., Tervonen, H., et al. (2019). Progress in cancer survival, mortality, and incidence in seven high-income countries 1995–2014 (ICBP SURVMARK-2): a population-based study. *The Lancet Oncology*, 20(11): 1493–505.

Arribas-Ayllon, M., Sarangi, S., and Clarke, A. (2011). Promissory accounts of personalisation in the commercialisation of genomic knowledge. *Communication & Medicine*, 8(1): 53–66.

Beaudevin, C., Peerbaye, A., and Bourgain, C. (2019). 'It has to become true genetics': tumour genetics and the division of diagnostic labour in the clinic. *Sociology of Health & Illness*, 41(4): 643–57.

Bekelman, J. E., and Joffe, S. (2018). Three steps toward a more sustainable path for targeted cancer drugs. *JAMA*, 319(21): 2167–8. doi:10.1001/jama.2018.3414.

Bell, K. (2009). 'If it almost kills you that means it's working!' Cultural models of chemotherapy expressed in a cancer support group. *Social Science & Medicine*, 68(1): 169–76.

Bell, K. (2013). Biomarkers, the molecular gaze and the transformation of cancer survivorship. *BioSocieties*, 8(2): 124–43.

Bell, K., and Kazanjian, A. (2011). PSA testing: molecular technologies and men's experience of prostate cancer survivorship. *Health, Risk & Society*, 13(2): 183–98.

Benjamin, R. (2014). Race for cures: rethinking the racial logics of 'trust' in biomedicine. *Sociology Compass*, 8(6): 755–69.

Benjamin, R. (2016). Informed refusal: toward a justice-based bioethics. *Science, Technology, & Human Values*, 41(6): 967–90.

Bickers, B., and Aukim-Hastie, C. (2009). New molecular biomarkers for the prognosis and management of prostate cancer – the post PSA era. *Anticancer Research*, 29(8): 3289–98.

Birch, K. (2017). Rethinking value in the bioeconomy: finance, assetization, and the management of value. *Science, Technology, & Human Values*, 42(3): 460–90.

Bodkin, H. (2018). Personalised medicine 'transforms' survival chances in incurable cancer. *The Telegraph*, 6 June, www.telegraph.co.uk/science/2018/06/05/personalised-medicine-transforms-survival-chances-incurable/ (accessed 8 July 2019).

Borad, M. J., and LoRusso, P. M. (2017). Twenty-first century precision medicine in oncology: genomic profiling in patients with cancer. *Mayo Clinic Proceedings*, 92(10): 1583–91.

Borup, M., Brown, N., Konrad, K., and Van Lente, H. (2006). The sociology of expectations in science and technology. *Technology Analysis & Strategic Management*, 18(3–4): 285–98.

Boseley, S. (2013). New breast cancer test could spare women chemotherapy. *The Guardian*, 26 September, https://www.theguardian.com/society/2013/sep/25/women-breast-cancer-test-spares-chemotherapy (accessed 20 June 2020).

Bourret, P., Keating, P., and Cambrosio, A. (2011). Regulating diagnosis in post-genomic medicine: re-aligning clinical judgement? *Social Science & Medicine*, 73(6): 816–24.

Braun, K., Moore, A., Herrmann, S. L., and Könninger, S. (2010). Science governance and the politics of proper talk: governmental bioethics as a new technology of reflexive government. *Economy and Society*, 39(4): 510–33.

Breast Cancer Now (2018). Breast Cancer Now responds to NICE decision to not to recommend use of tumour profiling tests. https://breastcancernow.org/news-and-blogs/news/nice-decide-not-to-recommend-use-of-tumour-profiling-tests (accessed 5 March 2018).

Brown, N., and Michael, M. (2003). A sociology of expectations: retrospecting prospects and prospecting retrospects. *Technology Analysis & Strategic Management*, 15(1): 3–18.

Brown, N., and Rappert, B. (2017). *Contested futures: a sociology of prospective techno-science*. Abingdon: Routledge.

Brown, P., and de Graaf, S. (2013). Considering a future which may not exist: the construction of time and expectations amidst advanced-stage cancer. *Health, Risk & Society*, 15(6–7): 543–60.

Brown, P., de Graaf, S., Hillen, M., Smets, E., and van Laarhoven, H. (2015). The interweaving of pharmaceutical and medical expectations as dynamics of micro-pharmaceuticalisation: advanced-stage cancer patients' hope in medicines alongside trust in professionals. *Social Science & Medicine*, 131: 313–21.

Brown, P., Hashem, F., and Calnan, M. (2016). Trust, regulatory processes and NICE decision-making: appraising cost-effectiveness models through appraising people and systems. *Social Studies of Science*, 46(1): 87–111.

Busfield, J. (2006). Pills, power, people: sociological understandings of the pharmaceutical industry. *Sociology*, 40(2): 297–314.

Callon, M., and Rabeharisoa, V. (2008). The growing engagement of emergent concerned groups in political and economic life: lessons from the French Association of Neuromuscular Disease Patients. *Science, Technology and Human Values*, 33: 230–61.

Cambrosio, A., Campbell, J., Keating, P., and Bourret, P. (2019). Multi-polar scripts: techno-regulatory environments and the rise of precision oncology diagnostic tests. *Social Science & Medicine* [online only/early view], 21 May 2019, 112317. https://doi.org/10.1016/j.socscimed.2019.05.022.

Cambrosio, A., Keating, P., Vignola-Gagné, E., Besle, S., and Bourret, P. (2018). Extending experimentation: oncology's fading boundary between research and care. *New Genetics and Society*, 37(3): 207–26.

Cancer Research UK (2014). Breast cancer survival statistics [online]. www.cancerresearchuk.org/health-professional/cancer-statistics/statistics-by-cancer-type/breast-cancer/survival (accessed 31 May 2019).

Chapple, A., Ziebland, S., and McPherson, A. (2004). Stigma, shame, and blame experienced by patients with lung cancer: qualitative study. *British Medical Journal*, 328(7454): 1470.

Chattoo, S., and Ahmad, W. I. U. (2003). The meaning of cancer: illness, biography and identity. In D. Kelleher and G. Leavey (eds), *Identity and Health*, 19–36. Abingdon: Routledge.

Clark, A. E., et al. (2003). Biomedicalization: technoscientific transformations of health, illness, and US biomedicine. *American Sociological Review*, 68(2): 161–94.

Cool, A. (2016). Detaching data from the state: biobanking and building big data in Sweden. *BioSocieties*, 11(3): 277–95.

Cooper, M. (2008). *Life as surplus: biotechnics and the transformations of capital*. Seattle, WA: Washington University Press.

Cooper, M., and Waldby, C. (2014). *Clinical labor: tissue donors and research subjects in the global bioeconomy*. Durham, NC: Duke University Press.

Corrigan, O. (2003). Empty ethics: the problem with informed consent. *Sociology of Health & Illness*, 25(7): 768–92.

Dabbs, D. J., Clark, B. Z., Serdy, K., Onisko, A., Brufsky, A. M., Smalley, S., Perkins, S. and Bhargava, R. (2018). Pathologist's health-care value in the triage of Oncotype DX® testing: a value-based pathology study of tumour biology with outcomes. *Histopathology*, 73(4): 692–700.

Davis, C. (2015). Drugs, cancer and end-of-life care: a case study of pharmaceuticalization? *Social Science & Medicine*, 131: 207–14.

Davis, C., and Abraham, J. (2013). *Unhealthy pharmaceutical regulation: innovation, politics and promissory science*. Basingstoke: Palgrave Macmillan.

Davies, S. C. (2017). *Annual Report of the Chief Medical Officer 2016, Generation Genome*. London: Department of Health.

Davies, M., and Sque, M. (2002). Living on the outside looking in: a theory of living with advanced breast cancer. *International Journal of Palliative Nursing*, 8(12): 583–90.

de Freitas, C., and Martin, G. (2015). Inclusive public participation in health: policy, practice and theoretical contributions to promote the involvement of marginalised groups in healthcare. *Social Science and Medicine*, 135: 31–9.

Degeling, C., Carter, S. M., and Rychetnik, L. (2015). Which public and why deliberate? A scoping review of public deliberation in public health and health policy research. *Social Science & Medicine*, 131: 114–21.

Derks, M. G., and van de Velde, C. J. (2018). Neoadjuvant chemotherapy in breast cancer: more than just downsizing. *The Lancet Oncology*, 19(1): 2–3.

DeVita, V. T., and Chu, E. (2008). A history of cancer chemotherapy. *Cancer Research*, 68(21): 8643–53.

Dheensa, S., Samuel, G., Lucassen, A. M., and Farsides, B. (2018). Towards a national genomics medicine service: the challenges facing clinical-research hybrid practices and the case of the 100,000 genomes project. *Journal of Medical Ethics*, 44(6): 397–403.

Dixon-Woods, M., Ashcroft, R. E., Jackson, C. J., Tobin, M. D., Kivits, J., Burton, P. R., and Samani, N. J. (2007). Beyond 'misunderstanding': written information and decisions about taking part in a genetic epidemiology study. *Social Science & Medicine*, 65(11): 2212–22.

Dixon-Woods, M., and Tarrant, C. (2009). Why do people cooperate with medical research? Findings from three studies. *Social Science & Medicine*, 68(12): 2215–22.

Dowsett, M., and Dunbier, A. K. (2008). Emerging biomarkers and new understanding of traditional markers in personalized therapy for breast cancer. *Clinical Cancer Research*, 14(24): 8019–26.

Dussauge, I., Claes-Fredrik, H., and Francis, L. (eds) (2015). *Value practices in the life sciences and medicine*. Oxford: Oxford University Press.

Ebeling, M. F. E. (2016). *Healthcare and big data: digital spectres and phantom objects*. Basingstoke: Palgrave.

Ehlers, N., and Krupar, S. (2014). Hope logics: biomedicine, affective conventions of cancer, and the governing of biocitizenry. *Configurations*, 22(3): 385–413.

Ehrenreich, B. (2001). Welcome to Cancerland: a mammogram leads to a cult of pink kitsch. *Harper's Magazine*, November, 43–53.

Felt, U., and Fochler, M. (2010). Machineries for making publics: inscribing and de-scribing publics in public engagement. *Minerva*, 48(3): 219–38.

Fojo, T., Mailankody, S., and Lo, A. (2014). Unintended consequences of expensive cancer therapeutics – the pursuit of marginal indications and a me-too mentality that stifles innovation and creativity. *JAMA Otolaryngology: Head & Neck Surgery*, 140(12): 1225–36. doi:10.1001/jamaoto.1570.

Fortun, M. (2008). *Promising genomics: Iceland and deCODE genetics in a world of speculation*. Berkeley, CA: University of California Press.

Frank, A. (2003). Survivorship as craft and conviction: reflections on research in progress. *Qualitative Health Research*, 13(2): 247–55.

Fujimura, J. H. (1996). *Crafting science: a sociohistory of the quest for the genetics of cancer*. Cambridge, MA: Harvard University Press.

Gabe, J., Chamberlain, K., Norris, P., Dew, K., Madden, H., and Hodgetts, D. (2012). The debate about the funding of Herceptin: a case study of 'countervailing powers'. *Social Science & Medicine*, 75(12): 2353–61.

Gallagher, J. (2018). Breast cancer: test means fewer women will need chemotherapy [online]. www.bbc.co.uk/news/health-44347381 (accessed 5 March 2019).

Gardner, J., Samuel, G., and Williams, C. (2015). Sociology of low expectations: recalibration as innovation work in biomedicine. *Science, Technology, & Human Values*, 40(6): 998–1021.

Gavan, S. P., Thompson, A. J., and Payne, K. (2018). The economic case for precision medicine. *Expert Review of Precision Medicine and Drug Development*, 3(1): 1–9.

Gerlitz, C., and Helmond, A. (2013). The like economy: social buttons and the data-intensive web. *New Media & Society*, 15(8): 1348–65.

Gillespie., C. (2012). The experience of risk as 'measured vulnerability': health screening and lay uses of numerical risk. *Sociology of Health & Illness*, 34(2): 194–207.

Good, M. J. D. (2001). The biotechnical embrace. *Culture, Medicine and Psychiatry*, 25(4): 395–410.

Good, M. J. D., Good, B. J., Schaffer, C., and Lind, S. E. (1990). American oncology and the discourse on hope. *Culture, Medicine and Psychiatry*, 14(1): 59–79.

Goven, J., and Pavone, V. (2015). The bioeconomy as political project: a Polanyian analysis. *Science, Technology, & Human Values*, 40(3): 302–37.

Greenhalgh, T. (2009). Patient and public involvement in chronic illness: beyond the expert patient. *British Medical Journal*, 338: b49.

Guy, M. (2019). Between 'going private' and 'NHS privatisation': patient choice, competition reforms and the relationship between the NHS and private healthcare in England. *Legal Studies*, 39(3): 479–98.

Haase, R., Michie, M., and Skinner, D. (2015). Flexible positions, managed hopes: the promissory bioeconomy of a whole genome sequencing cancer study. *Social Science & Medicine*, 130: 146–53.

Hall, S., Massey, D., and Rustin, M. (2014). After neoliberalism: analysing the present. In S. Hall, D. Massey and M. Rustin (eds), *After neoliberalism? The Kilburn manifesto*, 8–22. London: Lawrence & Wishart.

Ham, C., Baird, B., Gregory, S., Jabbal, J., and Alderwick, H. (2015). *The NHS under the coalition government. Part one: NHS reform*. London: The King's Fund. https://www.kingsfund.org.uk/sites/default/files/field/field_publication_file/the-nhs-under-the-coalition-government-part-one-nhs-reform.pdf (accessed 20 June 2020).

Hamilton, A. B. (1999). Psychological aspects of ovarian cancer. *Cancer Investigation*, 17(5): 335–41.

Hamilton, C. (2008). Intellectual property rights, the bioeconomy and the challenge of biopiracy. *Genomics, Society and Policy*, 4(3): 26.

Haraway, D. (1988). Situated knowledges: the science question in feminism and the privilege of partial perspective. *Feminist Studies*, 14(3): 575–99.

Harnan, S., Tappenden, P., Cooper, K., Stevens, J., Bessey, A., Rafia, R., Ward, S., Wong, R., Stein, R., and Brown, J. (2017). *Tumour profiling tests to guide adjuvant chemotherapy decisions in people with breast cancer (update of DG10). Technology Assessment Report: Final report to the National Institute for Health and Care Excellence*. Manchester: National Institute for Health and Care Excellence.

Harrison, C. J., Spencer, R. G., and Shackley, D. C. (2019). Transforming cancer outcomes in England: earlier and faster diagnoses, pathways to success, and empowering alliances. *Journal of Healthcare Leadership*, 11: 1–11.

Haslem, D. S., Chakravarty, I., Fulde, G., Gilbert, H., Tudor, B. P., Lin, K., Ford, J. M., and Nadauld, L. D. (2018). Precision oncology in advanced cancer patients improves overall survival with lower weekly healthcare costs. *Oncotarget*, 9(15): 12316–22.

Hayden, C. (2007). Taking as giving: bioscience, exchange, and the politics of benefit-sharing. *Social Studies of Science*, 37(5): 729–58.

Hedgecoe, A. (2004). *The politics of personalised medicine: pharmacogenetics in the clinic*. Cambridge: Cambridge University Press.

Hedgecoe, A. (2005). 'At the point at which you can do something about it, then it becomes more relevant': informed consent in the pharmacogenetic clinic. *Social Science & Medicine*, 61(6): 1201–10.

Hedgecoe, A., and Martin, P. (2003). The drugs don't work: expectations and the shaping of pharmacogenetics. *Social Studies of Science*, 33(3): 327–64.

Hiley, C. T., Le Quesne, J., Santis, G., Sharpe, R., De Castro, D. G., Middleton, G., and Swanton, C. (2016). Challenges in molecular testing in non-small-cell lung cancer patients with advanced disease. *The Lancet*, 388: 1002–11.

Hilgartner, S. (2017). *Reordering life: knowledge and control in the genomics revolution*. Cambridge, MA: MIT Press.

Hockings, E. (2014). Why we should opt out of the government's new patient database. *The Guardian*, 31 January, https://www.theguardian.com/science/political-science/2014/jan/31/why-we-should-opt-out-of-the-governments-new-patient-database (accessed 20 June 2020).

Hogarth, S., and Saukko, P. (2017). A market in the making: the past, present and future of direct-to-consumer genomics. *New Genetics and Society*, 36(3): 197–208.

Hood, L., and Auffray, C. (2013). Participatory medicine: a driving force for revolutionizing healthcare. *Genome Medicine*, 5: article no. 110.

Hood, L., and Friend, S. H. (2011). Predictive, personalized, preventive, participatory (P4) cancer medicine. *Nature Reviews Clinical Oncology*, 8(3): 184–7.

Horlick-Jones, T. (2011). Understanding fear of cancer recurrence in terms of damage to 'everyday health competence'. *Sociology of Health & Illness*, 33(6): 884–98.

Horst, M., and Irwin, A. (2010). Nations at ease with radical knowledge: on consensus, consensusing and false consensusness. *Social Studies of Science*, 40(1): 105–26.

Hubbard, G., Kidd, L., and Kearney, N. (2010). Disrupted lives and threats to identity: the experiences of people with colorectal cancer within the first year following diagnosis. *Health*, 14(2): 131–46.

Human Genomics Strategy Group (2012). *Building on our inheritance: genomic technology in healthcare*. London: Department of Health.

Interlandi, J. (2016). The paradox of precision medicine. *Scientific American*, 314(4): 24–5.

Jain, L. S. (2007). Living in prognosis: toward an elegiac politics. *Representations*, 98(1): 77–92.

Jain, L. S. (2013). *Malignant: how cancer becomes us*. Berkeley, CA: University of California Press.

James, N. (1992). Care = organisation + physical labour + emotional labour. *Sociology of Health & Illness*, 14(4): 488–509.

Jasanoff, S. (2015). Future imperfect: science, technology, and the imaginations of modernity. In S. Jasanoff and S-H. Kim (eds), *Dreamscapes of modernity: sociotechnical imaginaries and the fabrication of power*, 1–33. Chicago: University of Chicago Press.

Jasen, P. (2009). From the 'silent killer' to the 'whispering disease': ovarian cancer and the uses of metaphor. *Medical History*, 53(4): 489–512.

Jerolmack, C., and Tavory, I. (2014). Molds and totems: nonhumans and the constitution of the social self. *Sociological Theory*, 32(1): 64–77.

Joh, J. E., Esposito, N. N., Kiluk, J. V., Laronga, C., Lee, M. C., Loftus, L., Soliman, H., Boughey, J. C., Reynolds, C., Lawton, T. J., Acs, P. I., Gordan, L., and Acs, G. (2011). The effect of Oncotype DX recurrence score on treatment recommendations for patients with estrogen receptor-positive early stage breast cancer and correlation with estimation of recurrence risk by breast cancer specialists. *The Oncologist*, 16(11): 1520–6.

Kaiser, K. (2008). The meaning of the survivor identity for women with breast cancer. *Social Science & Medicine*, 67: 79–87.

Kaufman, S. R. (2015). *Ordinary medicine: extraordinary treatments, longer lives, and where to draw the line*. Durham, NC: Duke University Press.

Keating, P., and Cambrosio, A. (2011). *Cancer on trial: oncology as a new style of practice*. Chicago: University of Chicago Press.

Kerr, A., Swallow, J., Chekar, C. K., and Cunningham-Burley, S. (2019). Genomic research and the cancer clinic: uncertainty and expectations in professional accounts. *New Genetics and Society*, 38(2): 222–39.

Klawiter, M. (2004). Breast cancer in two regimes: the impact of social movements on illness experience. *Sociology of Health & Illness*, 26(6): 845–74.

Kohli-Laven, N., Bourret, P., Keating, P., and Cambrosio, A. (2011). Cancer clinical trials in the era of genomic signatures: biomedical innovation, clinical utility, and regulatory-scientific hybrids. *Social Studies of Science*, 41(4): 487–513.

Lamprell, K., Chin, M., and Braithwaite, J. (2018). The plot thickens: archetypal narrative structure in the melanoma patient journey. *Cogent Medicine*, 5(1): 1484053. https://doi.org/10.1080/2331205X.2018.1484053.

Landzelius, K. (2006). Introduction: patient organization movements and new metamorphoses in patienthood. *Social Science & Medicine*, 62(3): 529–37.

Largent, E. A., Fernandez Lynch, H., and McCoy, M. S. (2018). Patient-engaged research: choosing the 'right' patients to avoid pitfalls. *Hastings Center Report*, 48(5): 26–34.

Latimer, J., Featherstone, K., Atkinson, P., Clarke, A., Pilz, D. T., and Shaw, A. (2006). Rebirthing the clinic: the interaction of clinical judgment and genetic technology in the production of medical science. *Science, Technology, & Human Values*, 31(5): 599–630.

Lewin, S., and Reeves, S. (2011). Enacting 'team' and 'teamwork': using Goffman's theory of impression management to illuminate interprofessional practice on hospital wards. *Social Science & Medicine*, 72(10): 1595–602.

Lewis, S., Willis, K., Yee, J., and Kilbreath, S. (2016). Living well? Strategies used by women living with metastatic breast cancer. *Qualitative Health Research*, 26(9): 1167–79.

Light, D. W. (2010). Bearing the risks of prescription drugs. In D. W. Light (ed.), *The risks of prescription drugs*, 1–39. New York: Columbia University Press.

Llewellyn, H., Higgs, P., Sampson, E. L., Jones, L., and Thorne, L. (2018). Topographies of 'care pathways' and 'healthscapes': reconsidering the multiple journeys of people with a brain tumour. *Sociology of Health & Illness*, 40(3): 410–25.

Loncaster, J., Armstrong, A., Howell, S., Wilson, G., Welch, R., Chittalia, A., Valentine, W. J., and Bundred, N. J. (2017). Impact of Oncotype DX breast recurrence score testing on adjuvant chemotherapy use in early breast cancer: real world experience in Greater Manchester, UK. *European Journal of Surgical Oncology*, 43(5): 931–7.

Longo, D. L. (2013). Personalized cancer care is not new. *The Oncologist*, 18(6): 644–5.

Lupton, D. (2014). *Digital sociology*. Abingdon: Routledge.

MacKenzie, R., Chapman, S., Salkeld, G., and Holding, S. (2008). Media influence on Herceptin subsidization in Australia: application of the rule of rescue? *Journal of the Royal Society of Medicine*, 101(6): 305–12.

Madden, M., and Speed, E. (2017). Beware zombies and unicorns: toward critical patient and public involvement in health research in a neoliberal context. *Frontiers in Sociology*, 2: 7.

Madhu, N. (2017). Book review: Kaushik Sunder Rajan, *Pharmocracy: Value, Politics, and Knowledge in Global Medicine*. *Sociological Bulletin*, 66(3): 370–3.

Marcon, A. R., Bieber, M., and Caulfield, T. (2018). Representing a 'revolution': how the popular press has portrayed personalized medicine. *Genetics in Medicine*, 20(9): 950.

Marquart, J., Chen, E. Y., and Prasad, V. (2018). Estimation of the percentage of US patients with cancer who benefit from genome-driven oncology. *JAMA Oncology*, 4(8): 1093–8.

Martin, P. (2018). Genomic hope: promise in the bioeconomy. In S. Gibbon, B. Prainsack, S. Hilgartner and J. Lamoreaux (eds), *Routledge Handbook of Genomics, Health and Society*, 79–89. Abingdon: Routledge.

Matthews-King, A. (2018). Most women with early stage breast cancer can avoid toxic chemotherapy, major trial finds. *The Independent*, 3 June, https://www.independent.co.uk/news/health/breast-cancer-chemotherapy-genetic-test-hormone-therapy-survival-a8380906.html (accessed 20 June 2020).

Maughan, T. (2017). The promise and the hype of 'personalised medicine'. *The New Bioethics*, 23(1): 13–20.

McDonald, R., Waring, J., and Harrison, S. (2006). Rules, safety and the narrativisation of identity: a hospital operating theatre case study. *Sociology of Health & Illness*, 28(2): 178–202.

Mead, N., and Bower, P. (2000). Patient-centredness: a conceptual framework and review of the empirical literature. *Social Science & Medicine*, 51(7): 1087–110.

Medical Research Council (2014). Clinical trials: why multi-arms are better than two. [online]. www.insight.mrc.ac.uk/2014/07/25/clinical-trials-why-multi-arms-are-better-than-two/ (accessed 30 August 2018).

Merletti, F., Galassi, C., and Spadea, T. (2011). The socioeconomic determinants of cancer. *Environmental Health*, 10(1): S7.

Metzler, I. (2010). Biomarkers and their consequences for the biomedical profession: a social science perspective. *Personalized Medicine*, 7(4): 407–20.

Michael, M. (2012). 'What are we busy doing?' Engaging the idiot. *Science, Technology & Human Values*, 37(5): 528–54.

Michael, M. (2017a). Enacting Big Futures, Little Futures: toward an ecology of futures. *The Sociological Review*, 65(3): 509–24.

Michael, M. (2017b). Futures of the present: from performativity to prehension. In N. Brown and B. Rappert (eds), *Contested futures: a sociology of prospective techno-science*, 21–39. Abingdon: Routledge.

Middleton, G., Crack, L. R., Popat, S., Swanton, C., Hollingsworth, S. J., Buller, R., Walker, I., Carr, T. H., Wherton, D., and Billingham, L. J. (2015). The National Lung Matrix Trial: translating the biology of stratification in advanced non-small-cell lung cancer. *Annals of Oncology*, 26(12): 2464–9. https://doi.org/10.1093/annonc/mdv394.

Miles, D. W. (2001). Update on HER-2 as a target for cancer therapy Herceptin in the clinical setting. *Breast Cancer Research*, 3: 380–4.

Miller, F. A., Hayeems, R. Z., Bytautas, J. P., Bedard, P. L., Ernst, S., Hirte, H., Hotte, S., Oza, A., Razak, A., Welch, S., and Winquist, E. (2014). Testing personalized medicine: patient and physician expectations of next-generation genomic sequencing in late-stage cancer care. *European Journal of Human Genetics*, 22(3): 391.

Mitchell, R., and Waldby, C. (2010). National biobanks: clinical labor, risk production, and the creation of biovalue. *Science, Technology & Human Values*, 35(3): 330–55.

Montgomery, C. M. (2017a). Clinical trials and the drive to material standardisation: 'extending the rails' or reinventing the wheel? *Science and Technology Studies*, 30(4): 30–44.

Montgomery, C. M. (2017b). From standardization to adaptation: clinical trials and the moral economy of anticipation. *Science as Culture*, 26(2): 232–54.

Moore, D. A., Kushnir, M., Mak, G., Winter, H., Curiel, T., Voskoboynik, M., and Forster, M. (2019). Prospective analysis of 895 patients on a UK genomics review board. *ESMO Open*, 4(2): e000469.

Moorhead, J. (2018). No chemo: the test that made me a lucky breast cancer patient. *The Guardian*, 4 June, https://www.theguardian.com/commentisfree/2018/jun/04/chemo-breast-cancer-oncotype-dx-test (accessed 20 June 2020).

Morange, M. (1997). From the regulatory vision of cancer to the oncogene paradigm, 1975–1985. *Journal of the History of Biology*, 30(1): 1–29.

Moreira, T. (2011). Health care rationing in an age of uncertainty: a conceptual model. *Social Science & Medicine*, 72(8): 1333–41.

Murphy, M. (2012). *Seizing the means of reproduction: entanglements of feminism, health, and technoscience*. Durham, NC: Duke University Press.

Murphy, M. (2015). Unsettling care: troubling transnational itineraries of care in feminist health practices. *Social Studies of Science*, 45(5): 717–37.

Murphy, E., and Dingwall, R. (2007). Informed consent, anticipatory regulation and ethnographic practice. *Social Science & Medicine*, 65(11): 2223–34.

Nagaraj, G., and Ma, C. X. (2013). Adjuvant chemotherapy decisions in clinical practice for early-stage node-negative, estrogen receptor-positive, HER2-negative breast cancer: challenges and considerations, *Journal of the National Comprehensive Cancer Network*, 11(3): 246–51.

Nahuis, R., and Boon, W. P. C. (2011). The impact of patient advocacy: the case of innovative breast cancer drug reimbursement. *Sociology of Health & Illness*, 33(1): 1–15.

Nair, M., Sandhu, S. S., and Sharma, A. K. (2018). Cancer molecular markers: a guide to cancer detection and management. *Seminars in Cancer Biology*, 52: 39–55.

Nakagawa, H., and Fujita, M. (2018). Whole genome sequencing analysis for cancer genomics and precision medicine. *Cancer Science*, 109(3): 513–22.

Nawrocki, S. (2018). Molecular profiling of tumours for precision oncology – high hopes versus reality. *Contemporary Oncology*, 22(1A): 3.

Nelson, N. C., Keating, P., and Cambrosio, A. (2013). On being 'actionable': clinical sequencing and the emerging contours of a regime of genomic medicine in oncology. *New Genetics and Society*, 32(4): 405–28.

NICE (National Institute for Health and Care Excellence) (2013). Gene expression profiling and expanded immunohistochemistry tests for guiding adjuvant chemotherapy decisions in early breast cancer management: MammaPrint, Oncotype DX, IHC4 and Mammostrat. Manchester: National Institute for Health and Care Excellence.

NICE (National Institute for Health and Care Excellence) (2017). Tumour profiling tests to guide adjuvant chemotherapy decisions in people with breast cancer (update of DG10): Final Scope. Manchester: National Institute for Health and Care Excellence.

NICE (National Institute for Health and Care Excellence) (2018a). Diagnostics consultation document: tumour profiling tests to guide adjuvant chemotherapy decisions in early breast cancer. Manchester: National Institute for Health and Care Excellence.

NICE (National Institute for Health and Care Excellence) (2018b). Tumour profiling tests to guide adjuvant chemotherapy decisions in early breast cancer. Manchester: National Institute for Health and Care Excellence.

NICE (National Institute for Health and Care Excellence) (2018c). Tumour profiling tests to guide adjuvant chemotherapy decisions in early breast cancer: Diagnostics Consultation Document – Comments. Manchester: National Institute for Health and Care Excellence.

Novas, C. (2006). The political economy of hope: patients' organizations, science and biovalue. *BioSocieties*, 1(3): 289–305.

Nussinov, R., Hyunbum, J., Tsai, C.-J. and Cheng, F. (2019). Precision medicine and driver mutations: computational methods, functional assays and conformational principles for interpreting cancer drivers. *PLoS Computational Biology*, 15(3): e1006658.

Olopade, O. I., Grushko, T. A., Nanda, R. and Huo, D. (2008). Advances in breast cancer: pathways to personalized medicine. *Clinical Cancer Research*, 14(24): 7988–99.

Orgad, S. (2005). The transformative potential of online communication: the case of breast cancer patients' Internet spaces. *Feminist Media Studies*, 5(2): 141–61.

Parsons, E., and Atkinson, P. (1992). Lay constructions of genetic risk. *Sociology of Health & Illness*, 14(4): 437–55.

Petersen, A., and Lupton, D. (1997). *The new public health: health and self in the age of risk*. London: Sage.

Petersen, A., Schermuly, A. C., and Anderson, A. (2019). The shifting politics of patient activism: from bio-sociality to bio-digital citizenship. *Health*, 23(4): 478–94.

Powell, H. A. (2019). Socioeconomic deprivation and inequalities in lung cancer: time to delve deeper? *Thorax*, 74(1): 11–12.

Prainsack, B. (2017). *Personalized medicine: empowered patients in the 21st century?* New York: NYU Press.

Puig de La Bellacasa, M. P. (2011). Matters of care in technoscience: assembling neglected things. *Social Studies of Science*, 41(1): 85–106.

Puig de la Bellacasa, M. P. (2012). 'Nothing comes without its world': thinking with care. *The Sociological Review*, 60(2): 197–216.

Rabeharisoa, V., Moreira, T., and Akrich, M. (2014). Evidence-based activism: patients', users' and activists' groups in Knowledge Society. *Biosocieties*, 9(2): 111–28.

Rajan, K. S. (2006). *Biocapital: the constitution of postgenomic life*. Durham, NC: Duke University Press.

Rapp, R. (1998). Refusing prenatal diagnosis: the meanings of bioscience in a multicultural world. *Science, Technology, & Human Values*, 23(1): 45–70.

Roberts, K., and Clarke, C. (2009). Future disorientation following gynaeco-logical cancer: women's conceptualisation of risk after a life-threatening illness. *Health, Risk & Society*, 11(4): 353–66.

Rose, N. (2001). The politics of life itself. *Theory, Culture & Society*, 18(6): 1–30.

Ross, E., Swallow, J., Kerr, A., and Cunningham-Burley, S. (2019). Online accounts of gene expression profiling in early-stage breast cancer: interpreting genomic testing for chemotherapy decision making. *Health Expectations*, 22(1): 74–82.

Sample, I. (2014). PM: Genome project will transform cancer care. *The Guardian*, 1 August, www.theguardian.com/society/2014/aug/01/nhs-genetic-analysis-serious-diseases-diagnosed-treated (accessed 20 June 2020).

Samuel, G. N., and Farsides, B. (2017). The UK's 100,000 Genomes Project: manifesting policymakers' expectations. *New Genetics and Society*, 36(4): 336–53.

Schellekens, H., Aldosari, M., Talsma, H., and Mastrobattista, E. (2017). Making individualized drugs a reality. *Nature Biotechnology*, 35(6): 507–13.

Scottish Scientific Advisory Council (2019). *Informing the future of genomic medicine in Scotland*. Edinburgh: Scottish Science Advisory Council.

Selin, C. (2008). The sociology of the future: tracing stories of technology and time. *Sociology Compass*, 2(6): 1878–95.

Shack, L., Jordan, C., Thomson, C. S., Mak, V., and Møller, H. (2008). Variation in incidence of breast, lung and cervical cancer and malignant melanoma of skin by socioeconomic group in England. *BMC Cancer*, 8(1): 271.

Skloot, R. (2017). *The immortal life of Henrietta Lacks*. Portland, OR: Broadway Books.

Smyth, C. (2013). Test could spare women the ordeal of chemotherapy. *The Times*, 26 September, https://www.thetimes.co.uk/article/test-could-spare-women-the-ordeal-of-chemotherapy-b50tbbmmwf0 (accessed 20 June 2020).

Sparano, J. A., Gray, R. J., Makower, D. F., et al. (2018). Adjuvant chemotherapy guided by a 21-gene expression assay in breast cancer. *New England Journal of Medicine*, 379: 111–21.

Stage, C. (2017). *Networked cancer: affect, narrative and measurement*. Basingstoke: Palgrave Macmillan.

Star, S. L. (1985). Scientific work and uncertainty. *Social Studies of Science*, 15(3): 391–427.

Steinberg, D. L. (2015). The bad patient: estranged subjects of the cancer culture. *Body & Society*, 21(3): 115–43.

Suchman, L. (1996). Supporting articulation work. In R. Kling (ed.), *Computerization and controversy: value conflicts and social choices*, 407–23. London: Academic Press.

Sulik, G. (2009). Managing biomedical uncertainty: the technoscientific illness identity. *Sociology of Health & Illness*, 30(7): 1059–76.

Sulik, G. (2014). #Rethinkpink: moving beyond Breast Cancer Awareness SWS Distinguished Feminist Lecture. *Gender & Society*, 28(5): 655–78.

Swallow, J. (2019). Constructing classification boundaries in the memory clinic: negotiating risk and uncertainty in constituting mild cognitive impairment. *Sociology of Health & Illness* [online only/early view], 14 November 2019. https://doi.org/10.1111/1467-9566.1301.

Swallow, J., Kerr, A., Chekar, C. K., and Cunningham-Burley, S. (2020). Accomplishing an adaptive clinical trial for cancer: valuation practices and care work across the laboratory and the clinic. *Social Science & Medicine*, 252: 112949. https://doi.org/10.1016/j.socscimed.2020.112949

TallBear, K. (2013). *Native American DNA: tribal belonging and the false promise of genetic science*. Minneapolis, MN: University of Minnesota Press.

Tarkkala, H., Helén, I., and Snell, K. (2019). From health to wealth: the future of personalized medicine in the making. *Futures*, 109: 142–52.

Timmermans, S. (2005). From autonomy to accountability: the role of clinical practice guidelines in professional power. *Perspectives in Biology and Medicine*, 48(4): 490–501.

Tiriveedhi, V. (2018). Impact of precision medicine on drug repositioning and pricing: a too small to thrive crisis. *Journal of Personalized Medicine*, 8(4): 36. doi:10.3390/jpm8040036.

Tronto, J. C. (1993). *Moral boundaries: a political argument for an ethic of care*. London: Routledge.

Tupasela, A. (2017). Populations as brands in medical research: placing genes on the global genetic atlas. *BioSocieties*, 12(1): 47–65.

Tutton, R. (2012). Personalizing medicine: futures present and past. *Social Science & Medicine*, 75(10): 1721–8.

Tutton, R., and Jamie, K. (2013). Personalized medicine in context: social science perspectives. *Drug Discovery Today: Therapeutic Strategies*, 10(4): e183–e187.

Twigg, J., Wolkowitz, C., Cohen, R. L., and Nettleton, S. (2011). Conceptualising body work in health and social care. *Sociology of Health & Illness*, 33(2): 171–88.

Van Dijck, J., and Poell, T. (2013). Understanding social media logic. *Media and Communication*, 1(1): 2–14.

van Helvoort, T. (1999). A century of research into the cause of cancer: is the new oncogene paradigm revolutionary? *History and Philosophy of the Life Sciences*, 21(3): 293–330.

Van Lente, H., and Rip, A. (1998). The rise of membrane technology: from rhetorics to social reality. *Social Studies of Science*, 28(2): 221–54.

Vasella, D., and Slater, R. (2003). *Magic cancer bullet: how a tiny orange pill is rewriting medical history*. New York: Harper Business.

Vicari, S., and Cappai, F. (2016). Health activism and the logic of connective action: a case study of rare disease patient organisations. *Information, Communication & Society*, 19(11): 1653–71.

Ward, E., Jemal, A., Cokkinides, V., Singh, G. K., Cardinez, C., Ghafoor, A., and Thun, M. (2004). Cancer disparities by race/ethnicity and socioeconomic status. *CA: A Cancer Journal for Clinicians*, 54(2): 78–93.

Wenger, M. L., and Oliffe, L. J. (2014). Men managing cancer: a gender analysis. *Sociology of Health & Illness*, 36(1): 108–22.

West, H. J. (2017). Novel precision medicine trial designs umbrellas and baskets. *JAMA Oncology Patient*, 3(3): 423. doi:10.1001/jamaoncol.2016.5299.

Will, C., and Moreira, T. (2010). Medical proofs, social experiments. In C. Will and T. Moreira (eds), *Clinical trials in shifting contexts*. Aldershot: Ashgate.

Williams, S. J., Martin, P., and Gabe, J. (2011). The pharmaceuticalisation of society? A framework for analysis. *Sociology of Health & Illness*, 33(5): 710–25.

Yan, S. (2017). Prostate cancer patienthood in the genomic era: a study of patients' online accounts. Master of Public Health dissertation, University of Edinburgh.

Yeo, S. K., and Guan J.-L. (2017). Breast cancer: multiple subtypes within a tumor? *Trends in Cancer*, 3(1): 753–60.

Zafar, S. Y. (2015). Financial toxicity of cancer care: it's time to intervene. *Journal of the National Cancer Institute*, 108(5): djv370. doi:10.1093/jnci/djv370.

Ziebland, S., and Wyke, S. (2012). Health and illness in a connected world: how might sharing experiences on the internet affect people's health? *The Milbank Quarterly*, 90(2): 219–49.

Zuboff, S. (2019). *The age of surveillance capitalism: the fight for a human future at the new frontier of power*. London: Profile Books.

Index

100,000 Genomes Project 54, 119, 124, 152, 155–9, 164–5, 168–80, 223, 227, 237
23andMe 90

Abelson, J. 32
Abraham, J. 31, 65
access
  to participants for research 223–36
  to treatment as a patient 23, 246
Adam, B. 242–3
Adams, V. 23
adaptive trials 44–52, 118–25, 148, 245
advocacy 23, 31, 136, 208
ageing population 5
Agendia (company) 61
Aitman, Tim 156
Alectinib 198
algorithms 96–7
AstraZeneca (company) 122
austerity measures 5, 157
Avastin 36–7, 51, 184, 190–1, 203, 249

Bekelman, J. E. 186
Bell, Sir John 156
Bell, K. 42
benefit obtained from research 254–5
Benjamin, R. 212, 234, 237–8

Berg, Sancha 31
bioeconomy of genomic medicine 122, 154
'biomarketization' (Metzler) 91
biosociality 9, 249
blood cancer 119
Borad, M. J. 46
Bourret, P. 40
bowel cancer 191, 195
Braun, K. 162
breast cancer 29–35, 41, 58–64, 67, 119, 148, 188, 191, 223, 227, 239
  early-stage 76–85
Breast Cancer Now (charity) 64–5
Brexit 11, 155
British Medical Journal 198
Brown, N. 52–3
Brown, P. 47
Bully's Prize (game show) 110
'bureaucatic calculus' 186

Callon, M. 26–7
Cambrosio, A. 25–8, 32–3, 44–6, 118
Cameron, David 157–9, 167
Cameron, Ivan 158–9
campaigns for access to drugs 36–7
  see also media coverage and campaigns
'can do' attitude 244

Cancer Research UK (CRUK)
120–1, 124–5, 133, 186
cancer types 223
caring 241–55
blurred boundary with research
241, 254
forms of 244
at local level 244
on a macro scale 244
proliferation of 246
valuation of 243, 252
as work 245–6
central data repository 166
cervical cancer 36–7
charities and charitable donations
5–6, 185–6
chemotherapy 5, 59, 62–74,
77–86, 143, 188
China 155
clinical judgement 72
clinical trials 23–5, 118
clinical trials assistants (CTAs)
128–34, 227–8
clinicians
failure to participate in research
225–6
views on genomics 224–5
collaborative working 14
collective authorship 10
collective processes 248
Collins, P. A. 32
compassionate use of drugs 36,
187
complementary therapies 203–4
complexity of genomic medicine
185, 247
conditionality 115
Congenita (company) 154–5
consent process and consent forms
160–6, 169–81, 234, 238,
254
Corrigan, O. 161
cost considerations 23, 28, 74, 86
cost-effectiveness 23
crowdfunding 37, 51, 187–9,
197–209, 253

cultural capital 208
'cutting edge' treatments 251

Daily Mirror 198
data protection 176
Davies, Dame Sally 65
Davis, C. 38
day-to-day management of cancer
symptoms 115
deCODE (company) 154
de Graaf, S. 47
deprived groups and areas 5,
118–19
digital platforms 90, 189, 208–9
disappointment, management of
106–12
dosages 24, 27

economic benefits from new
treatments 250–1
embedding of new processes 119,
243
emotional labour 28, 106, 116,
206, 208, 226–7, 231–2, 253
empowerment 246
enthusiastic voices, privileging of
239
entrepreneurial approaches 250
'epistemological activism' 26, 30,
65
ethical approach to research 225,
238
ethical approval for research
223–5
ethnic minorities 221, 236–8
ethnographic research 14, 224
evidence-based practice 9, 24, 96
expectations, lowering of 119, 144
experimental value of trials 123
experimentation 185, 188, 198,
208, 241, 245, 250, 254
expert review groups 65
expertise
in challenging funding decisions
196–8, 208
new kinds of 250

Facebook 103, 176, 188, 194, 199–200, 204–5, 209
Farsides, B. 156
Felt, U. 212
feminism 7, 243
Finland 53–4
Fochler, M. 212
Food and Drug Administration (FDA) 27, 30, 41
foreshortened futures faced by some patients 99–100, 132, 148, 233
former patients' motivation for agreeing to be interviewed 218
Fortun, M. 154
Fox, Liam 155
Frank, A. 9, 189
Fujita, M. 52
funding of treatment 183–7
fundraising 188, 199, 203–8, 253
  hidden labour of 206
  success in 204–8
future patients, benefiting of 112, 131–2, 136, 147, 175, 248–9
future-crafting 7–9, 241–7, 251–2, 255

Gabe, J. 32–3
gastrointestinal tumours (GIST) 26–7
gatekeepers 223–7
gendered hierarchies in medicine 227
gene-expression profiling 41, 59–63, 66, 68, 73–5, 83
Genetech (company) 30–1
genomes 1–3, 14
Genomic Health (company) 59, 61, 88
Genomic Medicine Service 92, 180
genomic workers, solidarities between 255
Genomics England 154–7, 162–5, 237, 243

genomics (and genomic medicine) 22–3, 52–6, 75–6, 88, 115, 118–19, 126–7, 142, 152–8, 162–4, 170, 181, 214–15, 224–8, 234–9, 242–3, 247, 252–4
  clinicians' views on 224–5
  decentring of 252
  exaggerated expectations from 253
  institutionalisation and embedding of 243
  level of patients' understanding of 127, 235
  portrayal and auditing of 254
Gerlitz, C. 188
Gillespie, C. 43, 83–4
Gleevec 25–32, 35–7, 40
Good, M. J. D. 184
Google 176
gratitude, expressions of 253
Groves, C. 242–3
Guardian Health (company) 91
gynaecological cancers 88–116, 118, 148, 223

haematological cancers 171
Hamilton, A. B. 42
Hancock, Matt 124–5, 180
Haraway, D. 237
health inequalities 5, 214–15, 228, 237
Health and Social Care Act (2012) 159
Hedgecoe, A. 33–4, 68, 74
Helmond, A. 188
HER2 30–5
Herceptin 25, 30–7, 40, 46, 58, 68, 74
Hilgartner, S. 153–6, 164–5, 243
Hills, Dame Sue 180
hollowing-out of public services 5
hope, culture of 4
Horlick-Jones, T. 83
Horton, Richard 31
Human Genetics Commission 159

274   *Index*

Human Genome Project 59, 157, 164–5
Human Genomics Strategy Group 156
humour, deployment of 178

Iceland 154, 160
Illumina (company) 91, 157, 180
imagined communities 10
imatinib *see Gleevec*
incidence of cancer 5
incrementalism and incremental change 115, 125
infrastructures, organisational and environmental 14
innovation 9–10, 244
Instagram 188
Institute of Cancer Research 35
institutional structures 13
insurance schemes 189–90, 192
Interlandi, J. 55
involvement, extent of 23, 25, 51

Jain, L. S. 250–1, 255
Jardine, Lisa 31
Jeans, whose Genes? (film) 237–8
Jin Xiaotao 155
Joffe, S. 186

Kadcyla 36, 187
Kazanjian, A. 42
Keating, P. 25–8, 32–3, 45–6, 118
King's Fund 159

laboratories, workload of 227
Lamprell, K. 48
language barriers 221
Latimer, J. 72
life expectancy 186
Llewellyn, H. 51
LoRusso, P. M. 46
lung cancer 36, 118–22, 148, 223, 227, 249

McKinsey Global Institute 157
Macmillan nurses 220

MammaPrint 41, 61, 63
marginalised communities 236–7
marginalised patients 12–14
marketisation of genomic data 154
Matrix Trial 120–49
  totemic value of 143
Maughan, Tim 55
May, Theresa 155
media coverage and campaigns 31–3, 184, 208
metastatic cancer 102
Metzler, I. 89, 91
Michael, M. 9, 52–3, 212
middle-class bias 229–30, 236
Middleton, Gary 122
Mirati Therapeutics (company) 125
Mitchell, R. 53
molecular profiling 2, 22, 26, 39–44, 118, 241, 252, 255
  for advanced gynaecological cancer 88–116
'molecular turn' in cancer treatment 25, 33
monoclonal antibodies 25
Montgomery, C. M. 48, 149
Moorhead, Joanna 66
moral reflection 241
Moreira, T. 67
mortality rates 5

Nakagawa, H. 52
National Cancer Institute, US 30
National Health Service (NHS), UK 5–6, 31, 36, 53–4, 156–9, 181, 197–8, 207–8
  NHS Predict tool 69–70, 77, 80
National Institute for Health and Care Excellence (NICE), UK 31, 36, 60–8, 86, 94, 187, 191, 243
  Cancer Drugs Fund 184
Nelson, N. C. 41–2
neratinib 186
'niche-busters' 27

non-attendance at appointments 234
Novartis (company) 26

observation carried out for the present book 10
'oncogene paradigm' 24
Oncologica (company) 92
Oncotype DX 41, 60–3, 66–88, 92
optimisation of treatment 29, 52, 118, 149
optimism about prospects 241, 246
O'Shaughnessy, Lord 163
ovarian cancer 90, 103, 140
overtreatment 38

pancreatic cancer 225
Parker, Mike 159–60
participation in research 26, 212–13, 219–40
  accessing candidates for 223–36
  limitations of 212, 223, 231–4, 239
  misbehaviour in the course of 212–13
  obtaining value from 235, 251
  practicalities of 176
  reframed as obvious and routine 174–5
  see also patient participation; public engagement
partnerships between private companies and NHS clinicians 92
patient collectives 26
patient participation 171–80
  see also Public and Patient Involvement groups
patient pathways 185
personalisation of prognosis, prediction and diagnosis 39–44
personalised cancer medicine 1–7, 12–15, 22–4, 47, 54–6, 62,

68, 76, 87, 94, 97–8, 106, 118–21, 126, 147–50, 166–7, 174, 181, 183–7, 192, 195, 197, 211–13, 223–36, 239–46, 249–55
  delivery of 255
  difficulty of 167
  and holistic assessment of need 252
  linked with the wider bioeconomy 211–12
  origins of 23–4
  patients' responses to 28–9
  politics and economics of 255
  promise of 250, 253
personhood, *ordinary* and *educated* 180
Petersen, A. 188
petitioning by patients 26
P4 medicine 2, 211, 240
Pfizer (company) 122
pharmaceutical companies 29, 65–6, 127, 149, 180, 184–7, 207–8
Prainsack, B. 22–3
Prasad, Vinay 47
precision medicine 7, 120, 124, 186–7
Precision Medicine initiative (in the US) 22
pre-screening study (SMP2) for Matrix Trial 120–35, 139, 147
prevention of disease 5–6
pricing of drugs 27, 183, 187, 207
private healthcare 36, 38, 78, 92, 94, 98, 127, 187, 189–98, 249, 253
private patient units (PPUs) at NHS hospitals 192
professional status of clinicians 30
Prolaris 43
promissory scenarios 122, 240–1
promotional films 93

Prosigna (company) 60, 63, 67, 92
public engagement with research 236–9
Public and Patient Involvement groups for present study 2, 213–14, 236–7
Puig de la Bellacasa, M. P. 254

Rabeharisoa, V. 26–7
racism and racialisation 236–8
randomisation in trials 46
randomised controlled trials (RCTs) 94, 96, 100, 118
Rapp, R. 212
rare cancers 215, 223
reciprocity 248–9
recurrence risk 59, 62, 79–83, 101–2
'reflexive governance' (Braun *et al.*) 162
regional innovation funds 95
regulatory decision-making 67
relationship-building 222
remission 26, 28, 45
research governance 213
resilience 203
resistance to treatment 27, 246
resources, concern for *see* cost considerations
Rip, A. 24
Roche (company) 3–30, 156, 187

salience, lack of 112–14
Samuel, G. N. 156
Sapientia software 155
Schellekens, H. 186
science and technology studies (STS) 7, 12, 212, 247
scoping of personalised cancer medicine 213–22
Scottish Medicines Consortium 184
Scottish Scientific Advisory Council 43

self-funding *see* private healthcare
sense-making processes 248
Shannon, Kelly 50–1
shared understandings 247
SHIVA trial 45–7
Smith, Adam 155–6
smoking 118–19
social capital 148
social contract theory 6, 162
social media 90, 188, 197, 199, 204, 243
socio-economic circumstances 5
sociology of health and illness 9
speculative mono-futures, allure of 255
spending on cancer drugs 183
Stage, C. 200
Steinberg, D. L. 199, 250–1
Stevens, Simon 158
stigmatisation 118
stoicism 114
subtypes of cancer 2–3, 25, 29, 58, 249
Suchman, L. 126
Sullivan, Richard 186–7
survival rates 5, 59

'tailored' treatments 241
tamoxifen 218
targeted therapies 24–7, 44–5, 52, 92–3, 118–19, 122, 127, 147–8, 186–8, 196–7, 201, 203, 208, 252
    pricing of 183
    proliferation of 35–9
Tarkkala, H. 53
'theragnostics' 25
'therapeutic misconception' 160
transformative change 125, 164–71
Trial Assigning Individualised Options for Treatment (TAILORx) 66–7
trust 237–8
tumour growth 25

Tuskegee experiment 222
Tutton, R. 24

United States
  Centers for Disease Control and
    Prevention 183
  see also Food and Drug
    Administration; National
    Cancer Institute

valuation studies 9–10
van Lente, H. 24
Vasella, Dan 26
VGT study 100
Virtue (company pseudonym),
  promises of 103–6

Waldby, C. 53
Wellcome Trust 2, 157
whole-genome sequencing (WGS)
  52–4, 124, 150, 152, 157,
  180, 245
Windrush affair 238
women's cancers 223
working-class patients 229
worth of a life 253

Yorkshire and Humber Regional
  Genomics Service 237

Zuboff, S. 188

Lightning Source UK Ltd.
Milton Keynes UK
UKHW020915270221
379400UK00003B/183

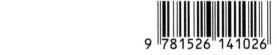